HESI: Workbook Containing 5 Full-Length Practice Tests

Phone: 800-496-5994

Email: info@smarteditionmedia.com

Library of Congress Cataloging-in-Publication Data
Smart Edition Media.

HESI Practice Test Workbook: 5 Full-Length Practice Tests/Smart Edition Media.

ISBN: 978-1-949147-63-6, 2nd edition.

1. HESI
2. Study Guides
3. Health Education Systems Incorporated
4. Nursing
5. Careers

Disclaimer:

The opinions expressed in this publication are the sole works of Smart Edition Media and were created independently from any National Evaluation Systems or other testing affiliates. Between the time of publication and printing, specific standards as well as testing formats and website information may change that are not included in part or in whole within this product. Smart Edition Media develops sample test questions, and they reflect similar content as on real tests; however, they are not former tests. Smart Edition Media assembles content that aligns with exam standards but makes no claims nor guarantees candidates a passing score.

Printed in the United States of America

HESI Practice Test Workbook: 5 Full-Length Practice Tests/Smart Edition Media.

ISBN: Print: 978-1-949147-63-6
      Ebook: 978-1-949147-64-3

Print and digital composition by Book Genesis, Inc.

HOW TO ACCESS THE ONLINE RESOURCES

To access your online resources, follow these instructions:

1. Go to www.smarteditionmedia.com.
2. Select Sign In in the website navigation at the top of the page .
3. Select your book.
4. Follow the instructions on the login page for locating the password in your book (the password is case sensitive, so be sure to include any capital letters at the beginning of the password).

 Practice tests

 Flashcards

 Videos

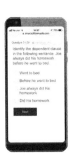

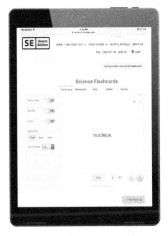

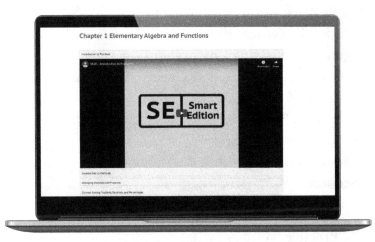

TABLE OF CONTENTS

INTRODUCTION

HESI Overview

The HESI Admissions Assessment Exam, or HESI A2, is an exam that is often selected by nursing schools and programs during the application process as a requirement for admissions. The test is taken by prospective students in order to assess their skills and abilities in areas such as English, math, and science.

There are other tests that are similar to the HESI exam, some of which may be required by your nursing program of choice. In addition, there are a total of 10 sections of the HESI exam that can be taken. Since every school utilizes the HESI differently, score requirements will also vary. Be sure to contact your school for their exact exam requirements before you begin the admissions process.

Entrance exams like the HESI help school administrators determine how a student is likely to perform in nursing school based on how well they perform during the first year in nursing school, as well as measure their outcome for success and completion of the nursing program. These tests also act as a preparation for the Registered Nurse licensure exam, the NCLEX, after graduation. The HESI specifically aims to prepare students for taking the NCLEX exam.

About This Book

This book provides you with an accurate and complete representation of the HESI Admissions Assessment Exam (HESI) and includes the core sections found on the exam: Math, Vocabulary and General Knowledge, Reading Comprehension, Grammar, Chemistry, Biology, Physics, and Anatomy & Physiology.

Online Sample Tests

The purchase of this book grants you access to two additional full-length practice tests online. You can locate these exams on the Smart Edition Media website. Go to the URL: https://smarteditionmedia.com/pages/hesiworkbook-online-resources and follow the password/login instructions.

HOW TO USE THIS BOOK

Congratulations in taking the first steps to achieving your career goals! Thank you for allowing Smart Edition Media to accompany you on your journey to success.

Taking practice tests is a great way to familiarize yourself with the test format, question structure, and content of an exam. Each of the tests in this workbook identifies the amount of time allowed for each section of the actual exam and includes questions similar to those you are likely to see on the actual exam. By using a methodical approach to taking practice tests, you can significantly improve your accuracy and comfortability with this exam.

Step One: Determine Your Baseline Score.

We suggest taking one of the online tests first as a diagnostic test. Log on to https://smarteditionmedia.com/pages/hesiworkbook-online-resources and follow the password/login instructions. Try to replicate actual test-taking conditions by working in a quiet location and adhering to the time limits of each section. Once you complete the text, you will receive a diagnostic report that will help you determine areas of strength and weakness.

Step Two: Practice Engaged Test-Taking Skills.

For your second and third practice test, use a printed test in this workbook. Simulate the same quiet environment, but allow yourself more time to take each section.

- Make margin notes of questions that you find challenging: circle unfamiliar words, use question marks or asterisks to note concepts that you want to review, and write reminders to yourself as you go through the test.
- Keep in mind the results of your diagnostic test as you work. If you need more time on a particular section, take it! If it helps you to look up words in a dictionary or refer to facts in a textbook or other reference book, by all means, do so! You can find helpful study tools, such as flashcards and subject-specific information sheets, at the online resources page of the Smart Edition Media website listed above.
- Check your answers against the Answer Key and read through the Answer Explanations for any question that you answered incorrectly, referring back to your reference materials for further clarification, if necessary.
- Note that the tests in this workbook are also available online. You can record your answers online even if you take the test in the book to receive the full diagnostic report. Simply log into the website and access the test to record your answers and run the analysis.

In these practice test scenarios, you should focus on completing as much as you can based on what you know and work through skills that might still be challenging by researching unfamiliar content as you go.

Step Three: Simulate the Actual Testing Environment.

Once you have taken a few practice tests and worked through your targeted areas of difficulty, it is time to simulate the actual testing environment.

- Schedule time with yourself to take the test as if it were the actual test day. Circle the date on your calendar and get a good night's rest the night before.
- Set aside a quiet place to take the test, clearing away all reference materials and notes. Eat a well-balanced meal or healthy snack before sitting down to take the test, just like you would the morning of the exam.
- Select one of the remaining full-length practice tests, in this workbook or online, and adhere to the time limits posted for each section as you take the test. Check your answers against the Answer Key and read through the Answer Explanations for any question that you answered incorrectly, referring back to your reference materials for further clarification, if necessary.
- Evaluate the results of your tests, from the first to the last one that you have taken. Acknowledge the improvements that you have made throughout this process, and note any trouble spots that remain. Use this information to target your remaining study time before the exam.
- By the time you have worked through this process, the date of your actual exam is most likely drawing near. If you have followed this outline, you will have at least one full-length practice test remaining. Use this test, either in sections or as a whole, as additional practice in the days preceding the actual test.
- Also note that you can use the results of this process—the margin notes that you've taken, the questions and your answers, and the Answer Explanations—can be used as a personalized study guide to keep the core skills sharp. Flip through your work the day before the exam to refresh your memory. You have put diligent, focused effort into preparing for this exam. Congratulations on all your hard work!

** This HESI A2 Workbook contains 5 full-length practice tests: three in the book (and online) and two exclusively online. These tests can be used alone or in conjunction with the HESI A2 Full Study Guide.

STUDY STRATEGIES AND TIPS

MAKE STUDY SESSIONS A PRIORITY

- Use a calendar to schedule your study sessions. Set aside a dedicated amount of time each day/week for studying. While it may seem difficult to manage given your other responsibilities, remember that to reach your goals, it is crucial to dedicate the time now to prepare for this test. A satisfactory score on your exam is the key to unlocking a multitude of opportunities for your future success.

- Do you work? Have children? Other obligations? Be sure to take these into account when creating your schedule. Work around them to ensure that your scheduled study sessions can be free of distractions.

> **TIPS FOR FINDING TIME TO STUDY.**
> - Wake up 1–2 hours before your family for some quiet time.
> - Study 1–2 hours before bedtime and after everything has quieted down.
> - Utilize weekends for longer study periods.
> - Hire a babysitter to watch children.

TAKE PRACTICE TESTS

- Smart Edition Media offers practice tests, both online and in print. Take as many as you can to help be prepared. This will eliminate any surprises you may encounter during the exam.

KNOW YOUR LEARNING STYLE

- Identify your strengths and weaknesses as a student. All students are different and everyone has a different learning style. Do not compare yourself to others.

- Howard Gardner, a developmental psychologist at Harvard University, has studied the ways in which people learn new information. He has identified seven distinct intelligences. According to his theory:

"we are all able to know the world through language, logical-mathematical analysis, spatial representation, musical thinking, the use of the body to solve problems or to make things, an understanding of other individuals, and an understanding of ourselves. Where individuals differ is in the strength of these intelligences - the so-called profile of intelligences -and in the ways in which such intelligences are invoked and combined to carry out different tasks, solve diverse problems, and progress in various domains."

- Knowing your learning style can help you to tailor your studying efforts to suit your natural strengths.

- What ways help you learn best? Videos? Reading textbooks? Find the best way for you to study and learn/review the material.

WHAT IS YOUR LEARNING STYLE?

- **Visual-Spatial** – Do you like to draw, do jigsaw puzzles, read maps, daydream? Creating drawings, graphic organizers, or watching videos might be useful for you.
- **Bodily-kinesthetic** – Do you like movement, making things, physical activity? Do you communicate well through body language or like to be taught through physical activity? Hands-on learning, acting out, and role playing are tools you might try.
- **Musical** – Do you show sensitivity to rhythm and sound? If you love music and are also sensitive to sounds in your environments, it might be beneficial to study with music in the background. You can turn lessons into lyricsor speak rhythmically to aid in content retention.
- **Interpersonal** – Do you have many friends, empathy for others, street smarts, and interact well with others? You might learn best in a group setting. Form a study group with other students who are preparing for the same exam. Technology makes it easy to connect—if you are unable to meet in person, teleconferencing or video chats are useful tools to aid interpersonal learners in connecting with others.
- **Intrapersonal** – Do you prefer to work alone than in a group? Are you in tune with your inner feelings? Do you follow your intuition and possess a strong will, confidence and opinions? Independent study and introspection will be ideal for you. Reading books, using creative materials, and keeping a diary of your progress will be helpful. Intrapersonal learners are the most independent of the learners.
- **Linguistic** – Do you use words effectively, have highly developed auditory skills, and often think in words? Do you like reading, playing word games, making up poetry or stories? Learning tools such as computers, games, and multimedia will be beneficial to your studies.
- **Logical-Mathematical** – Do you think conceptually, abstractly, and are able to see and explore patterns and relationships? Try exploring subject matter through logic games, experiments, and puzzles.

CREATE THE OPTIMAL STUDY ENVIRONMENT

- Some people enjoy listening to soft background music when they study. (Instrumental music is a good choice.) Others need to have a silent space in order to concentrate. Which do you prefer? Either way, it is best to create an environment that is free of distractions for your study sessions.
- Have study guide – Will travel! Leave your house; daily routines and chores can be distractions. Check out your local library, a coffee shop, or another quiet space to remove yourself from distractions and daunting household tasks that compete for your attention.
- Create a Technology-Free Zone. Silence the ringer on your cell phone and place it out of reach to prevent surfing the Web, social media interactions, and email/texting exchanges. Turn off the television, radio, or other devices while you study.
- Are you comfy? Find a comfortable, but not *too* comfortable, place to study. Sit at a desk or table in a straight, upright chair. Avoid sitting on the couch, a bed, or in front of the TV. Wear clothing that is not binding and restricting.
- Keep your area organized. Have all the materials you need available and ready: Smart Edition study guide, computer, notebook, pen, calculator, and pencil/eraser. Use a desk lamp or overhead light that provides ample lighting to prevent eyestrain and fatigue.

HEALTHY BODY, HEALTHY MIND

- Consider these words of wisdom from Buddha, "To keep the body in good health is a duty – otherwise we shall not be able to keep our mind strong and clear."

KEYS TO CREATING A HEALTHY BODY AND MIND:

- Drink water – Stay hydrated! Limit drinks with excessive sugar or caffeine.
- Eat natural foods – Make smart food choices and avoid greasy, fatty, sugary foods.
- Think positively – You can do this! Do not doubt yourself, and trust in the process.
- Exercise daily – If you have a workout routine, stick to it! If you are more sedentary, now is a great time to begin! Try yoga or a low-impact sport. Simply walking at a brisk pace will help to get your heart rate going.
- Sleep well – Getting a good night's sleep is important, but too few of us actually make it a priority. Aim to get eight hours of uninterrupted sleep in order to maximize your mental focus, memory, learning, and physical wellbeing.

FINAL THOUGHTS

- Remember to relax and take breaks during study sessions.
- Review the testing material. Go over topics you already know for a refresher.
- Focus more time on less familiar subjects.

EXAM PREPARATION

In addition to studying for your upcoming exam, it is important to keep in mind that you need to prepare your mind and body as well. When preparing to take an exam as a whole, not just studying, taking practice exams, and reviewing math rules—it is critical to prepare your body in order to be mentally and physically ready. Often, your success rate will be much higher when you are *fully* ready.

Here are some tips to keep in mind when preparing for your exam:

SEVERAL WEEKS/DAYS BEFORE THE EXAM

- Get a full night of sleep, approximately 8 hours.
- Turn off electronics before bed.
- Exercise regularly.
- Eat a healthy balanced diet, including fruits and vegetables.
- Drink water.

THE NIGHT BEFORE

- Eat a good dinner.
- Pack materials/bag, healthy snacks, and water.

- Gather materials you need for the test: your ID and receipt of test. You do not want to be scrambling the morning of the exam. If you are unsure of what to bring with you, check with your testing center or test administrator.
- Map the location of test center, and identify how you will be getting there (driving, public transportation, uber, etc.), when you need to leave, and parking options.
- Lay your clothes out. Wear comfortable clothes and shoes, and do not wear items that are too hot/cold.
- Allow minimum of ~8 hours of sleep.
- Avoid coffee and alcohol.
- Do not take any medications or drugs to help you sleep.
- Set alarm.

THE DAY OF THE EXAM

- Wake up early, allowing ample time to do all the things you need to do and for travel.
- Eat a healthy, well-rounded breakfast.
- Drink water.
- Leave early and arrive early, and leave time for any traffic or any other unforeseeable circumstances.
- Arrive early and check in for the exam. This will give you enough time to relax, take off your coat, and become comfortable with your surroundings.

Take a deep breath, get ready, go! You got this!

FREQUENTLY ASKED QUESTIONS

Test dates

- The test may be offered every few weeks.
- Check with you nursing school/program on when/if they administer the test

How to register for the HESI exam

- Go to the EVOLVE main website and choose *I'm a Student*
- Choose *Register for Distance Testing, Register, Redeem/Checkout*
- You will then make an Evolve account, read registered user agreement, Choose *Yes, I accept, SUBMIT*
- Once you have registered, you will be able to access My Content under the *HESI Assessment Student Access* link
- Select *Payments*: Here you will be able to choose test date and location
- Follow the prompts and *Proceed to Checkout*
- Price: $35-70. The cost will vary among the school/testing center administering the test

Where do I take the test?

- The test is administered by many nursing schools or community colleges.
- May be able to take it at a testing center
- Check with your school/program of choice for available dates and locations
- Many schools/programs will offer the test in accordance to the application due dates.

How long is the test?

- The time of the test will vary based on how many sections you are required to take.
- 4 hours is the allotted time for the entire test
- Must be completed in one testing session
- Arrive 30 minutes early to allow for check-in

What subjects are on the test?

- Test subjects and admission criteria will vary amongst programs. Check with your nursing school/program about which section they require.
- Test subjects may include: Math, Vocabulary and general knowledge, Reading Comprehension, Grammar, Chemistry, Biology, Physics, Anatomy & Physiology
- Your school may also require a Learning Style/Personality Profile exam

How many questions are on the test?

- This will vary according to test subjects required

How long does it take to get the test score?

- You will receive your score immediately once you have completed the exam

What if I fail the test?

- You may be able to retake the test; however, the test is only offered.
- Check with your program/school for their requirements on retesting
- There may be a waiting period for retaking the test

How long are scores valid?

- Check with your nursing program for this information

What to bring/not bring to the test?

BRING:

- Government Issued Photo ID (Driver's license, Passport, Green card)
- Receipt of payment of the test OR payment for test (if not paid for in advance)
- Login information (Username and Password)
- You will need to create an account when registering for the test.

DO NOT BRING:

- Books or study material
- Calculator (one will be provided to you)
- Electronics of any kind (cell/smart phone, digital/smart watches, beepers/pagers, tablet)
- Food or Drink

HESI VS NCLEX...WHAT'S THE DIFFERENCE?

Upon finishing nursing school, all students must sit for the nursing licensure exam, NCLEX, in order to become a registered nurse (RN) and to become licensed to practice nursing in your state.

The HESI is known to be a predictor or practice exam to prepare students for the NCLEX. Schools may require HESI for entrance into the nursing program but may also be used as a mid-curricular exam (to see how well a student is being prepared), or an exit exam (at the end of nursing school, to identify their preparedness to take the NCLEX).

Some schools may require the HESI exit exam in order to graduate. Just remember, all school are different and have different requirements when it comes to the HESI. But, if you do have to take it, consider yourself lucky as you will be adequately prepared when you sit for the NCLEX.

In conclusion, in order to become a licensed RN, everyone MUST take the NCLEX. The HESI is generally only required as either an entrance exam into nursing school or an exit exam.

Schools that require the HESI will vary.

HESI PRACTICE EXAM 1

SECTION I. MATHEMATICS

You have 50 minutes to complete 50 questions.

1. What is the difference between natural numbers and whole numbers?

   A. They are the same.

   B. The whole numbers include zero, but the natural numbers exclude zero.

   C. The natural numbers only go to 10, but the whole numbers have no limit.

   D. The whole numbers include negative numbers, but the natural numbers do not.

2. What is 1,078 + 0?

   A. 1,078

   B. 1,079

   C. 2,156

   D. None of the above

3. How many millimeters are in a measurement that is 4 centimeters, 3 meters, and 7 millimeters long? (Note that a centimeter is 10 millimeters and a meter is 1,000 millimeters.)

   A. 347

   B. 437

   C. 3,047

   D. 3,407

4. Evaluate the expression 8 – 27.

   A. –35

   B. –19

   C. 0

   D. 19

5. Which sequence is in the correct order from least to greatest?

   A. –10, 0, 1, 8

   B. 0, 1, 8 –10

   C. –10, 8, 1, 0

   D. 8, 1, 0, –10

6. Which statement best describes a remainder in division?

   A. The quotient minus the divisor

   B. The product of the dividend and divisor

   C. The difference between the dividend and the quotient

   D. The portion of a dividend not evenly divisible by the divisor

7. What is 96 ÷ 12?

   A. 8

   B. 84

   C. 960

   D. 1,152

8. Evaluate the expression 12 ÷ 4 × 3 + 1.

   A. 0

   B. 2

   C. 10

   D. 12

9. Evaluate the expression 28 × 43.

   A. 71

   B. 196

   C. 1,204

   D. 1,960

10. Which statement about positive and negative numbers is true?

    A. The product of two negative numbers is negative.

    B. The product of two negative numbers is positive.

    C. The product of two negative numbers is zero.

    D. None of the above.

11. Change $0.\overline{63}$ to a fraction. Simplify completely.

   A. $\frac{5}{9}$

   B. $\frac{7}{11}$

   C. $\frac{2}{3}$

   D. $\frac{5}{6}$

12. Which fraction is the greatest?

   A. $\frac{5}{12}$

   B. $\frac{1}{3}$

   C. $\frac{1}{6}$

   D. $\frac{1}{4}$

13. Which decimal is the greatest?

   A. 4.04

   B. 4.404

   C. 4.44

   D. 4.044

14. Which decimal is the least?

   A. 0.786

   B. 0.876

   C. 0.687

   D. 0.768

15. Multiply $\frac{2}{3} \times \frac{4}{15}$.

   A. $\frac{3}{20}$

   B. $\frac{1}{6}$

   C. $\frac{8}{45}$

   D. $\frac{1}{3}$

16. Multiply $\frac{3}{16} \times \frac{4}{7}$.

   A. $\frac{3}{28}$

   B. $\frac{1}{9}$

   C. $\frac{1}{6}$

   D. $\frac{7}{9}$

17. Divide $\frac{1}{10} \div \frac{2}{3}$.

   A. $\frac{1}{15}$

   B. $\frac{1}{10}$

   C. $\frac{3}{20}$

   D. $\frac{3}{5}$

18. Divide $\frac{8}{9} \div \frac{5}{7}$.

   A. $\frac{11}{45}$

   B. $\frac{40}{63}$

   C. $1\frac{11}{45}$

   D. $1\frac{40}{63}$

19. Which proportion yields a number for the unknown that is different from the others?

   A. $\frac{13}{75} = \frac{158}{?}$

   B. $\frac{75}{13} = \frac{?}{158}$

   C. $\frac{158}{?} = \frac{13}{75}$

   D. $\frac{75}{13} = \frac{158}{?}$

20. If 35% of a cattle herd is Ayrshire and the rest is Jersey, and it has 195 Jerseys, how many cattle are in the herd?

   A. 230

   B. 263

   C. 300

   D. 557

21. Which number satisfies the proportion $\frac{378}{?} = \frac{18}{7}$?

   A. 18

   B. 147

   C. 972

   D. 2,646

22. If 15 out of every 250 contest entries are winners, what percentage of entries are winners?

   A. 0.06%

   B. 6%

   C. 15%

   D. 17%

23. Which percent is equal to the ratio 4:5?

   A. 44%

   B. 45%

   C. 80%

   D. 125%

24. Convert 2.5 miles to feet.

   A. 2,112 feet

   B. 2,640 feet

   C. 10,560 feet

   D. 13,200 feet

25. Convert 147 liters to kiloliters.

   A. 0.147 kiloliters

   B. 1.47 kiloliters

   C. 1,470 kiloliters

   D. 147,000 kiloliters

26. Convert 48 inches to yards.

   A. $1\frac{1}{3}$ yards

   B. 4 yards

   C. $4\frac{4}{5}$ yards

   D. 16 yards

27. Convert 18 meters to millimeters.

   A. 180 millimeters

   B. 1,800 millimeters

   C. 18,000 millimeters

   D. 180,000 millimeters

28. Identify 1435 in 12-hour clock time.

    A. 12:35 a.m.   C. 12:35 p.m.

    B. 2:35 a.m.   D. 2:35 p.m.

29. Solve the equation for the unknown, $\frac{c}{-4} = -12$.

    A. -16 C. 3

    B. -8 D. 48

30. Solve the inequality for the unknown, $3(x + 1) + 2(x + 1) \geq 5(3-x) + 4(x + 2)$.

    A. $x \geq 0$ C. $x \geq 2$

    B. $x \geq 1$ D. $x \geq 3$

31. Solve the inequality for the unknown, $\frac{1}{4}x - \frac{1}{3}(x + 2) \leq \frac{1}{12}(2x + 3) + x - 1$.

    A. $x \leq -\frac{1}{15}$ C. $x \leq \frac{1}{15}$

    B. $x \geq -\frac{1}{15}$ D. $x \geq \frac{1}{15}$

32. Solve the equation for the unknown, $-6d = 36$.

    A. -216 C. 30

    B. -6 D. 42

33. Solve the system of equations,
$x = -3y + 10$
$x = 3y - 8$

    A. $(-1, 3)$ C. $(1, 3)$

    B. $(-3, 1)$ D. $(3, 1)$

34. Solve the system of equations, $\begin{matrix} y = -4x - 4 \\ y = -5x - 4 \end{matrix}$.

    A. $(0, -4)$ C. $(0, 4)$

    B. $(-4, 0)$ D. $(4, 0)$

35. Solve the system of equations, $\begin{matrix} x = -y - 7 \\ -x + 4y = 22 \end{matrix}$.

    A. $(10, -3)$ C. $(5, 7)$

    B. $(-10, 3)$ D. $(7, 5)$

36. In a word game, a player loses 8 points when using an invalid word. If there were 65 invalid words, how many points were lost during the game?

    A. -520 C. -73

    B. -480 D. -57

37. In a game, positive and negative points can be scored. For 10 turns, the point total is $-5, +4, -7, -2, 0, +3, +5, -6, -4, +2$. What is the average point total?

    A. -2 C. 1

    B. -1 D. 2

38. In a state, the highest elevation is 1,450 feet and the lowest elevation is -80 feet. What is the difference in the elevations in feet?

    A. $1,370$ C. $1,530$

    B. $1,430$ D. $1,570$

39. A business reported a loss on Monday and Tuesday of $300 each day, a loss on Wednesday of $100, a profit on Thursday of $400, and a profit on Friday and Saturday for $600 each day. What was the total profit or loss for the week?

    A. $600   C. $1,400

    B. $900   D. $2,300

40. One athlete had a salary of about 3×10^7 dollars per year and another athlete had a salary of about 2×10^6 dollars per year. How many times larger is the salary of the first athlete?

    A. 2 C. 10

    B. 5 D. 15

41. Simplify $(4x^3)^2$.

    A. $8x^5$ C. $16x^5$

    B. $8x^6$ D. $16x^6$

42. Solve the system of equations by graphing, $y = \frac{1}{3}x + 2$
$y = \frac{2}{3}x + 5$.

A.

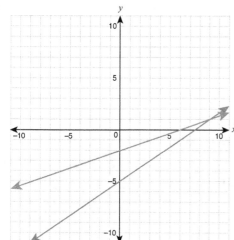

C.

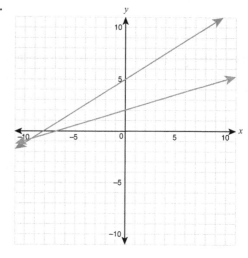

B.

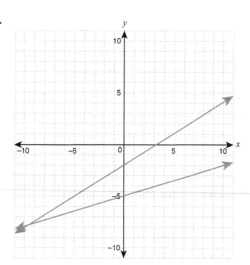

D.

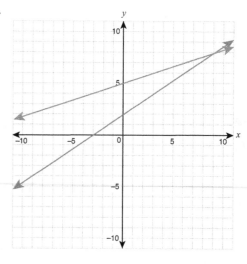

43. Solve $x^2 = 225$.

   A. $-5, 5$ C. $-15, 15$

   B. $-10, 10$ D. $-20, 20$

44. Simplify $(6^3)^{-1}$.

   A. $\frac{1}{216}$ C. 18

   B. $\frac{1}{18}$ D. 216

45. Solve $x^2 = 81$.

   A. $-6, 6$ C. $-8, 8$

   B. $-7, 7$ D. $-9, 9$

46. Apply the polynomial identity to rewrite $x^3 + 125$.

   A. $(x + 5)(x^2 - 5x + 25)$

   B. $(x - 5)(x^2 - 10x + 25)$

   C. $(x + 5)(x^2 + 5x + 25)$

   D. $(x - 5)(x^2 + 10x + 25)$

47. Multiply, $2xy(-3xy + x^2y^2)$.

   A. $-6x^2y^2 + 2x^3y^3$

   B. $-6xy + 2x^2y^2$

   C. $-6x^2y^2 + 2x^2y^2$

   D. $-6xy - 8x^3y^3$

48. Solve the system of equations by graphing, $\begin{array}{l} y = -2x + 3 \\ y = 3 \end{array}$.

A.

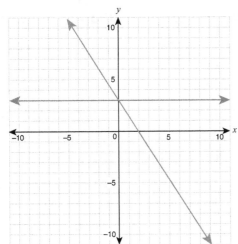

C.

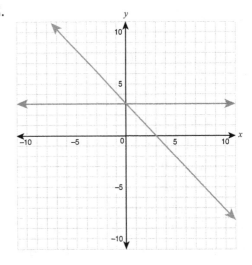

B.

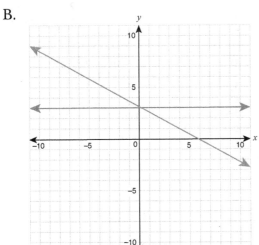

D.

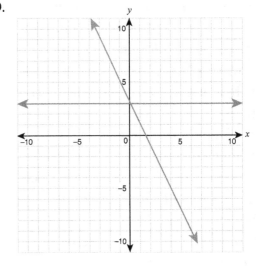

49. Apply the polynomial identity to rewrite
$x^2 + 20x + 100$.

A. $x^2 + 100$ C. $(x^2 + 10)^2$

B. $(x + 10)^2$ D. $(10x)^2$

50. Perform the operation,
$(6x^2 + 3xy - 5y^2) - (4x^2 - 2xy + 6y^2)$.

A. $2x^2 + xy - 11xy^2$

B. $2x^2 + xy + xy^2$

C. $2x^2 + 5xy - 11y^2$

D. $2x^2 + 5xy + xy^2$

SECTION II. READING COMPREHENSION

You have 50 minutes to complete 47 questions.

Please read the text below and answer questions 1-5.

Most people have had the pleasure of tasting a delicious chocolate chip cookie at some point in their lives. But what most folks do not know is that chocolate chip cookies were invented by accident. Ruth Graves Wakefield, owner of the popular Toll House Inn in Whitman, Massachusetts, prepared all the food for her guests. People came from all over to stay at the Toll House Inn and eat her famous Chocolate Butter Drop Do cookies. These chocolate cookies were such a hit that Ruth found herself baking them on a daily basis. One day, when she was preparing the recipe, she realized she had run out of baker's chocolate. She decided to break up a block of Nestle semi-sweet chocolate instead, expecting them to melt and disperse through the cookie dough. To her surprise, when she took the cookies out of the oven, the chocolate morsels retained their shape as "chips" in the cookie, thereby making them the first batch of chocolate chip cookies every baked. Ruth's chocolate chip cookies were so popular that they ended up permanently replacing her Chocolate Butter Drop Do cookies. Thanks to this happy accident, people all over the world get to enjoy one of the best desserts ever invented!

1. **Which sentence is the topic sentence?**
   A. Most people have had the pleasure of tasting a delicious chocolate chip cookie at some point in their lives.
   B. But what most folks do not know is that chocolate chip cookies were invented by accident.
   C. She decided to break up a block of Nestle semi-sweet chocolate instead, expecting them to melt and disperse through the cookie dough.
   D. Ruth's chocolate chip cookies were so popular that they ended up permanently replacing her Chocolate Butter Drop Do cookies.

2. **In the paragraph, the chocolate chip cookie is:**
   A. the topic.
   B. the main idea.
   C. a supporting detail.
   D. the topic sentence.

3. **Which sentence summarizes the main idea of the paragraph?**
   A. Chocolate chip cookies are more popular than Chocolate Butter Drop Do cookies.
   B. Ruth Graves Wakefield became famous for her chocolate chip cookie recipe.
   C. One of the most classic and popular desserts came about unexpectedly.
   D. It takes a whole lot of work to create something long-lasting.

4. **Which of the following sentences from the paragraph is a supporting detail of the topic sentence?**

   A. Ruth Graves Wakefield, owner of the popular Toll House Inn in Whitman, Massachusetts, prepared all the food for her guests on a daily basis.

   B. People came from all over to stay at the Toll House Inn and eat her famous Chocolate Butter Drop Do cookies.

   C. These chocolate cookies were such a hit that Ruth found herself baking them on a daily basis.

   D. She decided to break up a block of Nestle semi-sweet chocolate instead, expecting them to melt and disperse through the cookie dough.

5. **Which sentence would *best* function as a supporting detail in this paragraph?**

   A. The Nestle Company now owns the rights to Ruth Graves Wakefield's chocolate chip cookie recipe.

   B. Ruth Graves Wakefield tasted the cookies with the chocolate morsels in them and realized immediately how delicious they were.

   C. Today people buy pre-packaged chocolate chips instead of breaking off pieces of chocolate from a Nestle bar.

   D. Ruth Graves Wakefield sold her recipe in exchange for a lifetime of free chocolate.

Please read the text below and answer questions 6-8.

In the past 10-15 years, koalas have been repeatedly harmed or killed in traffic accidents. When the animals cross busy roads, highways, and intersections to get to their food source, the eucalyptus tree, many of them meet a terrible fate. Australian developers have been taking over koala habitats to keep up with the country's booming population. This has resulted in the endangerment of the country's most beloved animal. Concerned individuals have taken action by creating koala "pathways," routes traveling over roads, highways, and intersections to ensure koalas keep safe. In addition, koala hospitals have been established in these areas to rehabilitate the injured animals.

6. **Which phrase best describes the topic of the group of sentences above?**

   A. An analysis of animal behavior in the wild

   B. An account of human impact on an animal species

   C. A description of a building development plan

   D. An examination of the ways humans help animals

7. **Which of the following sentences would best function as a topic sentence to unite the information in the paragraph?**

   A. Over 4,000 koalas are hurt or injured each year by automobiles.

   B. Koalas spend most of their time in trees but need to occasionally travel across roads to move around.

   C. Human encroachment on natural habitats has negatively impacted the koala population.

   D. Australia's building development projects have tripled over the past decade.

8. **Which sentence provides another supporting detail to address the topic of the sentences above?**

   A. Kangaroos, emus, and wombats are other popular animals in Australia.

   B. Australia has a diverse population of citizens from various countries throughout the world.

   C. Koalas are not bears but marsupials, mammals that carry their young in a pouch.

   D. Australia has erected over 500 koala pathways over the past two years.

9. **Which graphic would best support a paragraph about the different parts of a car engine and their functions?**

   A. Diagram   C. Bar Graph

   B. Flowchart   D. Pie Chart

10. **Which graphic would best support a paragraph explaining the percentage breakdowns of how a charity organization plans to spend a large donation?**

    A. Diagram   C. Bar Graph

    B. Flowchart   D. Pie Chart

Read the following text and its summary and answer questions 11-12.

Text: In the late 1800s, life was terrible for some children. The Industrial Revolution was in full effect and factories sprang up in urban areas all over the country. Many innocent children left the comforts of home for the big cities to make money for their families. Children as young as 6 were forced to work long hours with dangerous equipment for little pay. A lot of children grew ill or even died on the job. Factory owners justified this abominable treatment by claiming they fed, clothed, and provided shelter for these children.

Summary: The author argues that children led awful lives during the Industrial Revolution due to long work hours, dangerous equipment, and little pay. Factory owners justified this treatment even though children were becoming ill or dying.

11. **Is this summary effective? Why or why not?**

    A. The summary is effective because it captures the emotional component of the text.

    B. The summary is effective because it restates the key points in a new way.

    C. The summary is ineffective because it makes its own claims and judgments.

    D. The summary is ineffective because it is structurally the same as the original.

12. **If the first line of the summary were replaced, which of the following lines would make the summary ineffective?**

    A. The author claims that in the late 1800s, life was terrible for some children.

    B. The author states that during the Industrial Revolution, children faced many hardships.

    C. The author claims that life was difficult for children during the Industrial Revolution.

    D. The author states that children who worked during the Industrial Revolution had it tough.

Read the following text and then answer questions 13-15.

Preheat your oven to 350 degrees. Get out all your equipment and ingredients. In a large bowl, combine flour, baking powder, sugar, and salt. Then soften 1 cup of butter. Next add the butter and the eggs to the dry mixture and stir until all the ingredients are mixed. Mix in the chocolate chips. Using a tablespoon, spoon out the batter onto a pre-greased cookie sheet. Bake in the oven for 12 minutes. Allow cookies to cool before serving.

13. **Which of the following words from the text indicate sequence?**

    A. Preheat, Mix   C. Using, Bake

    B. Then, Next   D. Get, In

14. **What does the term "pre-greased cookie sheet" tell you?**

    A. That you are supposed to grease the cookie sheet right after you spoon out the batter

    B. That you are supposed to grease the cookie sheet at some time before putting the batter onto it

    C. That you are supposed to grease the cookie sheet after preheating the oven

    D. That you are supposed to grease the cookie sheet after the baking the cookies

15. **What sequence word would best fit at the beginning of this sentence from the text?**

    Allow cookies to cool before serving.

    A. Then   C. After

    B. Last   D. Next

16. **Read the sentences below.**

Jose is a determined individual. _____ he spent five days trying to teach himself the guitar since he wants to join a band. _____ his mom claims that he exhibited similar behavior when he wanted to walk; he spent hours getting up and falling down.

Which words or phrases should be inserted into the blanks to provide clear transitions between these ideas?

A. In conclusion; Thus

B. First; Consequently

C. Although; In contrast

D. For instance; Moreover

17. **Read the sentences below.**

Dogs are typically friendly, loyal animals that love people. <u>However</u>, some people train their dogs to be vicious fighters, so you should always ask pet owners if it's safe to approach their dog.

What is the function of the <u>underlined</u> transition word in sentence two?

A. To express a contrast

B. To provide an example

C. To add emphasis to a point

D. To indicate time or sequence

18. **Which word functions as a transition in the sentence below?**

Cassandra loved reading and writing books as a child. Thus she became an English teacher in her adult life.

A. Loved

B. Child

C. Thus

D. Became

19. **Which word functions as a transition in the sentences below?**

However you celebrate the holidays, it's time to spend with your family. It's also a time to enjoy some good food!

A. However

B. Time

C. Also

D. Some

Read the passage and answer questions 20-23.

Dear Mr. O'Hara,

I am writing to let you know how much of a positive impact you have made on our daughter. Before being in your algebra class, Violet was math phobic. She would shut down when new concepts would not come to her easily. As a result, she did not pass many tests. Despite this past struggle, she has blossomed in your class! Your patience and dedication have made all the difference in the world. Above all, your one-on-one sessions with her have truly helped her in ways you cannot imagine. She is a more confident and capable math student, thanks to you. We cannot thank you enough.

Fondly,

Bridgette Foster

20. **Which adjective best describes the tone of this passage?**

A. Arrogant

B. Hopeless

C. Friendly

D. Appreciative

21. **Which phrase from the passage has an openly appreciative and warm tone?**

A. I am writing to let you now

B. you have made on our daughter

C. made all the difference

D. We cannot thank you enough

22. What mood would this passage most likely evoke in the math teacher, Mr. O'Hara?

   A. Calm

   B. Grateful

   C. Sympathetic

   D. Embarrassment

23. Which transition word or phrase from the passage adds emphasis to the writer's point?

   A. Being   C. Despite

   B. As a result   D. Above all

24. An author's purpose is the:

   A. opinion the author has on a topic.

   B. reason an author writes something.

   C. strategies the author uses to entertain.

   D. details the author uses to explain a process.

25. What is the most likely purpose of a cookbook full of Mediterranean recipes?

   A. To decide   C. To persuade

   B. To inform   D. To entertain

26. What is the most likely purpose of an article explaining why Eastern medicine is better than Western medicine?

   A. To decide   C. To persuade

   B. To inform   D. To entertain

27. What is the most likely purpose of a realistic fiction book about one family's experience living in a foreign country?

   A. To decide   C. To persuade

   B. To inform   D. To entertain

Read the passages below and answer questions 28-31.

Many people find termites to be destructive little pests, but they are actually ingenious little creatures. If you were to look at a termite mound, you would see firsthand how incredible these insects are.

These masters of construction work together to erect high-functioning, green-energy skyscrapers out of nothing but soil, saliva, and dung. The largest one documented is in the Democratic Republic of the Congo. This mound, measuring 12.8 meters (41.9 feet) tall, has heat regulation and air conditioning systems. It also contains numerous chambers for food storage, gardens, and babies.

And just think: a termite is only .6 cm long, yet it is still capable of building a sophisticated structure that's 2,013 times its size!

*

As we hiked along the dusty trail deep within the Congo, four tour guide suddenly stopped and held up his hand.

Panic rose inside me, as I expected to see a ghastly hyena or other vicious predator in our midst. But he slowly pointed toward a large mound off the side of the path.

What on earth?

It rose high above us, a tall, sandy structure, its arms outstretched to the sky.

"This," he began in a whisper so as not to disturb its inhabitants, "is a termite mound. Inside are thousands of termites.

These tiny little insects have worked together to build this massive structure. And not only is it ventilated to keep them cool, but there are tons of little rooms or chambers inside for different purposes."

WHOA. A termite mound? How on earth did those pesky little bugs do that?

28. **What is the purpose of the first paragraph of Passage 1?**

    A. To inform
    B. To distract
    C. To persuade
    D. To entertain

29. **What is the primary purpose of Passage 2?**

    A. To inform
    B. To distract
    C. To persuade
    D. To entertain

30. **With which statement would the author of Passage 1 most likely agree?**

    A. Things are not always what they seem.

    B. The best things in life come in small packages.

    C. If you try hard enough, you can achieve anything.

    D. Working together accomplishes more than working alone.

31. **The author of Passage 1 supports his/her points primarily by:**

    A. telling humanizing stories.

    B. relying on facts and logic.

    C. pointing to expert sources.

    D. using fear tactics and manipulation.

Read the following paragraphs and answer questions 32-35.

The idea of getting rid of homework at the elementary school level is debatable, but giving young children a well-needed break after school is undoubtedly beneficial. A study of elementary age children and homework showed that daily homework causes high rates of anxiety and depression in young people. In contrast, schools that have gotten rid of the homework requirement have reported a drop in depression and anxiety among students.

According to a nationwide analysis of standardized testing scores, schools that have gotten rid of homework have seen benefits. Test scores have gone up incrementally from year to year. On the contrary, schools that mandate daily homework have seen stagnant test scores. Therefore, it is safe to say that homework does nothing to enhance student learning at all.

32. **Which statement expresses an opinion?**

    A. The idea of getting rid of homework at the elementary school level is debatable, but giving young children a well-needed break after school is undoubtedly beneficial.

    B. A study of elementary age children and homework showed that daily homework causes high rates of anxiety and depression in young people.

    C. In contrast, schools that have gotten rid of the homework requirement have reported a drop in depression and anxiety among students.

    D. According to a nationwide analysis of standardized testing scores, schools that have gotten rid of homework have seen benefits.

33. **Consider the following sentence from the passage:**

    On the contrary, schools that mandate daily homework have seen stagnant test scores.

    Is this statement a fact or an opinion? Why?

    A. An opinion because it focuses on the beliefs of the schools involved

    B. An opinion because it expresses how the author feels about standardized test scores

    C. A fact because it shares test score results, which are something that can be verified

    D. A fact because it relies on the schools' projected test score results

34. **What is the primary argument of the passage?**

    A. Schools need to change the type of homework they give to elementary school students.

    B. There are no clear benefits from giving elementary-aged students daily homework.

    C. A school's standardized test scores is a good measure of how the school is performing overall.

    D. Schools with stagnant test scores would benefit from giving students more homework.

35. **Which sentence in the passage displays faulty reasoning?**

    A. According to a nationwide analysis of standardized testing scores, schools that have gotten rid of homework have seen benefits.

    B. Test scores have gone up incrementally from year to year.

    C. On the contrary, schools that mandate daily homework have seen stagnant test scores.

    D. Therefore, it is safe to say that homework does nothing to enhance student learning at all.

Read the following passage and answer questions 36-40.

Most children under the age of 18 are very overweight. Statistics show that 1 in 3 children have been diagnosed as obese. This is way too much. There is no reason for so many children to be obese. Children must eat a balanced diet devoid of processed foods, get at least one hour of exercise every day, and make sure to sleep for 9-10 hours or suffer a life full of health problems. It is concerning to see so many unhealthy young people in our country. Children should be active and engaged instead of sedentary and apathetic.

36. **What is the primary argument in the passage?**

    A. A healthy diet is the key to a healthy life.

    B. Childhood obesity is a major problem in our country.

    C. Too many young people do not get enough sleep each night.

    D. Processed foods have caused too much obesity in our youth.

37. **Which excerpt from the text, if true, is a fact?**

    A. Most children under the age of 18 are very overweight.

    B. Statistics show that 1 in 3 children have been diagnosed as obese.

    C. It is concerning to see so many unhealthy young people in our country.

    D. Children should be active and engaged instead of sedentary and apathetic.

38. **Re-read the following sentence from the passage:**

    Children must eat a balanced diet devoid of processed foods, get at least one hour of exercise every day, and make sure to sleep for 9-10 hours or suffer a life full of health problems.

    What type of faulty reasoning does this sentence display?

    A. Either/or fallacy

    B. Circular reasoning

    C. Bandwagon argument

    D. False statement of cause and effect

39. **Re-read the following sentence from the passage:**

    There is no reason for so many children to be obese.

    The reasoning in this sentence is faulty because it:

    A. suggests that this is an issue that needs attention.

    B. claims that there are many ways to solve this problem.

    C. restates the argument in different words instead of providing evidence.

    D. assumes that children are overweight based on their own choices.

40. Re-read the following sentence from the passage:

Most children under the age of 18 are very overweight.

This sentence is an opinion because it:

A. reflects a belief, not a verifiable fact.

B. does not say how much "very" is.

C. restricts its statement to children under 18.

D. lumps all people under 18 into one category.

41. **Which of the following is an example of a primary source?**

A. An encyclopedia

B. A biography

C. A guidebook

D. An interview

42. **What type of source is an online video presentation on the works of a famous artist?**

A. Primary

B. Secondary

C. Tertiary

D. None of the above

43. **Which source would provide the *least* credible information to a researcher interested in studying changes in parenting techniques over the past forty years?**

A. An op-ed piece in today's newspaper on the hardships of being a parent of an adolescent

B. A currently published interview with a pediatrician on the benefits of positive discipline

C. A book published in 1985 about best practices in raising your child

D. A recent article in *Parenting Magazine* about parenting in the 1980s vs. today

44. **Which of the following is *not* a primary source on Betty Friedan?**

A. An interview with Betty Friedan

B. *The Feminine Mystique* by Betty Friedan

C. A speech Betty Friedan gave during a march

D. An article about Betty Friedan's contributions to the women's movement

Study the infographic below and answer questions 45-46.

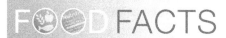 FACTS

Safe Food Handling: Four Simple Steps

 CLEAN   SEPARATE   COOK   CHILL

CLEAN
Wash hands and surfaces often

- Wash your hands with warm water and soap for at least 20 seconds before and after handling food and after using the bathroom, changing diapers, and handling pets.
- Wash your cutting boards, dishes, utensils, and counter tops with hot soapy water after preparing each food item.
- Consider using paper towels to clean up kitchen surfaces. If you use cloth towels, launder them often in the hot cycle.
- Rinse fresh fruits and vegetables under running tap water, including those with skins and rinds that are not eaten. Scrub firm produce with a clean produce brush.
- With canned goods, remember to clean lids before opening.

SEPARATE
Separate raw meats from other foods

- Separate raw meat, poultry, seafood, and eggs from other foods in your grocery shopping cart, grocery bags, and refrigerator.
- Use one cutting board for fresh produce and a separate one for raw meat, poultry, and seafood.
- Never place cooked food on a plate that previously held raw meat, poultry, seafood, or eggs unless the plate has been washed in hot, soapy water.
- Don't reuse marinades used on raw foods unless you bring them to a boil first.

COOK
Cook to the right temperature

- Color and texture are unreliable indicators of safety. Using a food thermometer is the only way to ensure the safety of meat, poultry, seafood, and egg products for all cooking methods. These foods must be cooked to a safe minimum internal temperature to destroy any harmful bacteria.
- Cook eggs until the yolk and white are firm. Only use recipes in which eggs are cooked or heated thoroughly.
- When cooking in a microwave oven, cover food, stir, and rotate for even cooking. If there is no turntable, rotate the dish by hand once or twice during cooking. Always allow standing time, which completes the cooking, before checking the internal temperature with a food thermometer.
- Bring sauces, soups and gravy to a boil when reheating.

CHILL
Refrigerate foods promptly

- Use an appliance thermometer to be sure the temperature is consistently 40° F or below and the freezer temperature is 0° F or below.
- Refrigerate or freeze meat, poultry, eggs, seafood, and other perishables within 2 hours of cooking or purchasing. Refrigerate within 1 hour if the temperature outside is above 90° F.
- Never thaw food at room temperature, such as on the counter top. There are three safe ways to defrost food: in the refrigerator, in cold water, and in the microwave. Food thawed in cold water or in the microwave should be cooked immediately.
- Always marinate food in the refrigerator.
- Divide large amounts of leftovers into shallow containers for quicker cooling in the refrigerator.

April 2017 4

For more information, contact the U.S. Food and Drug Administration, Center for Food Safety and Applied Nutrition's Food and Cosmetic Information Center at **1-888-SAFEFOOD** (toll free), Monday through Friday 10 AM to 4 PM ET (except Thursdays from 12:30 PM to 1:30 PM ET and Federal holidays). Or, visit the FDA website at **http://www.fda.gov/educationresourcelibrary**

Resource: The Food and Drug Administration

45. **Which of the following is a sign that the infographic is credible?**

   A. The information is presented in an organized way.

   B. The information comes from a government agency.

   C. The information is colorful and engaging.

   D. The information has the word "FACTS" written at the top.

46. **What could a skeptical reader do to verify the facts on the infographic?**

   A. Interview one chef from a local restaurant about safe food handling

   B. Contact the agencies whose phone numbers are listed at the bottom of the page

   C. Check a tertiary source like Wikipedia to verify the information

   D. Compare the infographic's information about safe food handling to a cook's blog

47. **An art major finds a video presentation of a group of people commenting on the works of a famous artist she has been studying. She is deciding if it is a credible source. Which detail about the video, if true, would *not* give her reason to trust the video?**

   A. The video was filmed within the past two years.

   B. One of the speakers is a renowned Ivy League Art History professor.

   C. Real paintings of the artist's work are shown.

   D. The video is highly edited and some speakers are cut off mid-sentence.

SECTION III. VOCABULARY & GENERAL KNOWLEDGE

You have 50 minutes to complete 50 questions.

1. What is the best definition of the word *spherical*?

   A. Hard
   B. Round
   C. Rough
   D. Absorbent

2. Which of the following root words means "old"?

   A. mort
   B. dorm
   C. rupt
   D. veter

3. What is the best definition of the word *endotherm*?

   A. A plant-eating animal
   B. A meat-eating animal
   C. A cold-blooded animal
   D. A warm-blooded animal

4. Which of the following suffixes means "more"?

   A. -er
   B. -ed
   C. -en
   D. -es

5. Which of the following root words means "truth"?

   A. viv
   B. ver
   C. voc
   D. vac

6. Which of the following prefixes means "false"?

   A. con-
   B. non-
   C. trans-
   D. pseudo-

7. The use of the prefix tri- in the word tripod indicates what about a stand?

   A. It has 1 leg
   B. It has 2 legs
   C. It has 3 legs
   D. It has 4 legs

8. *Fallible* most nearly means capable of

   A. falling down.
   B. making errors.
   C. being dishonest.
   D. talking loudly.

9. Select the meaning of the underlined word in the sentence.

   The man studies extraterrestrial beings.

   A. Ones that are not of this earth
   B. Ones that are similar to humans
   C. Ones that live in tropical habitats
   D. Ones that live high in the mountains

10. What is the best definition of the word synchronize?

    A. To cause to occur at a later time
    B. To cause to occur at different times
    C. To cause to occur at an earlier time
    D. To cause to occur at the same time

11. Which of the following suffixes means "younger" or "inferior"?

    A. -ling
    B. -loger
    C. -opsy
    D. -tude

12. Which of the following root words means "self"?

    A. dem
    B. bio
    C. bene
    D. auto

13. Which of the following prefixes means "between"?

    A. homo-
    B. intra-
    C. epi-
    D. fore-

14. **Select the word from the following sentence that has more than one meaning.**

Phillip watched excitedly as the racecars sped around the track.

   A. excitedly   C. racecars

   B. watched   D. track

15. **Select the correct definition of the underlined word that has multiple meanings in the sentence.**

The loud crack of thunder frightened the children.

   A. Space   C. Joke

   B. Bang   D. Attempt

16. **Select the context clue from the following sentence that helps you define the multiple meaning word court.**

The emperor's court was a dedicated group that accompanied him on many of his excursions.

   A. "dedicated"   C. "accompanied"

   B. "group"   D. "excursions"

17. **Select the meaning of the underlined word in the sentence based on the context clues.**

According to Greek mythology, Zeus is an omnipotent god who has the power to do just about anything he wants to mortals and other gods.

   A. Almighty   C. Respected

   B. Vindictive   D. Generous

18. **Select the context clue from the following sentence that helps you define the word ornate.**

The silverware at the dinner party was quite ornate, and people admired the detail in the candlelight.

   A. "silverware"   C. "detail"

   B. "party"   D. "candlelight"

19. **Select the word from the following sentence that has more than one meaning.**

The excited parents spent a lot of time decorating their newborn's nursery.

   A. excited   C. decorating

   B. parents   D. nursery

20. **Select the correct definition of the underlined word that has multiple meanings in the sentence.**

Juanita was excited that her newly published book received a glowing review.

   A. Critique   C. Inspection

   B. Periodical   D. Appraisal

21. **Select the context clue from the following sentence that helps you define the multiple meaning word spring.**

As a child, Kerry would always spring out of bed to see what present her parents left her on the kitchen table.

   A. "child"   C. "to see"

   B. "out of"   D. "present"

22. **Select the meaning of the underlined word in the sentence based on the context clues.**

    Toddlers can be quite <u>petulant</u> when they don't get their way, often resorting to tears and tantrums.

    A. Unkind   C. Irritable

    B. Spoiled   D. Disobedient

23. **Select the context clue from the following sentence that helps you define the word <u>prohibit</u>.**

    In the 1920s, the government decided to prohibit alcohol, and people were forbidden to drink at home or in public places.

    A. "alcohol"   C. "drink"

    B. "forbidden"   D. "places"

24. **Select the word from the following sentence that has more than one meaning.**

    Since the young boy was a minor, he was not allowed to watch the R-rated movie.

    A. young   C. allowed

    B. minor   D. movie

25. **Select the correct definition of the underlined word that has more than one meaning in the sentence.**

    The television was not receiving a <u>signal</u>, so the family could not watch the Academy Awards.

    A. A sign   C. A piece of evidence

    B. A gesture   D. An electrical impulse

26. **Select the context clue from the following sentence that helps you define the multiple meaning word <u>jerk</u>.**

    I have such contempt for my brother when he acts like a <u>jerk</u> in front of my friends.

    A. "contempt"   C. "acts"

    B. "brother"   D. "friends"

27. **Select the meaning of the underlined word in the sentence based on the context clues.**

    The high school English teacher was known to <u>scorn</u> those who did not use proper grammar.

    A. Deride   C. Support

    B. Teach   D. Harass

28. **Select the context clue from the following sentence that helps you define the word <u>ubiquitous</u>.**

    Cell phones are ubiquitous these days and are commonly seen in even the most remote parts of the world.

    A. "these days"   C. "most remote"

    B. "commonly seen" D. "parts of"

29. **Select the word from the following sentence that has more than one meaning.**

    Sheldon is a master chess player who competes in tournaments all over the world.

    A. master   C. competes

    B. chess   D. tournaments

30. Select the correct definition of the underlined word that has more than one meaning in the sentence.

Molly went into the gas station to see if they would break a twenty-dollar bill.

A. Shatter   C. Get change

B. Fracture   D. Make a pause

31. Select the meaning of the underlined word in the sentence based on the context clues.

The flowers began to flourish after getting plenty of sunshine and water.

A. Wilt   C. Smell

B. Grow   D. Disappear

32. Select the context clue from the following sentence that helps you define the multiple meaning word scale.

The criminals tried to scale a fence, but they got stuck and ended up getting nabbed by the police.

A. "criminals"   C. "stuck"

B. "fence"   D. "police"

33. Select the meaning of the underlined word in the sentence based on the context clues.

Stanley was pleasantly surprised when he saw the interest his savings account had earned over the years.

A. Profit   C. Concern

B. Stake   D. Attentiveness

34. Select the meaning of the underlined word in the sentence based on the context clues.

The woman was hired because she was competent, having successfully tackled many IT problems at her previous job.

A. Skilled   C. Outgoing

B. Generous   D. Industrious

35. Which of the following root words means "hearing"?

A. Angi   C. Audi

B. Aden   D. Aort

36. In this sentence, the root indicates that the doctor will surgically repair which body part?

The surgeon was getting ready to perform an osteoplasty.

A. A bone   C. A kidney

B. An eye   D. An ear

37. Based on your knowledge of medical roots, prefixes, and suffixes, which of the following words means "the study and treatment of tumors"?

A. Radiology   C. Cardiology

B. Oncology   D. Neurology

38. Which of the following suffixes means "weakness"?

A. -asthenia   C. -dynia

B. -centesis   D. -ectomy

39. Based on your knowledge of roots, prefixes, and suffixes, what is a hysterectomy?

A. Repair of a hernia   C. Treatment of an infection

B. Removal of the uterus   D. Exploration of the stomach

40. Adding which of the following suffixes to pelvi- , from the word pelvis, would show that the pelvis's dimensions are being measured?

    A. -pathy
    B. -ology
    C. –algia
    D. -metry

41. Look at the following sentence.

    The young boy had a pulmonary issue and had to be seen by the doctor right away.

    What kind of issue was the boy having?

    A. An issue with his throat
    B. An issue with his lungs
    C. An issue with his pelvis
    D. An issue with his heart

42. Read the following sentence.

    After surgery, the patient began to experience rhinalgia and needed pain medication.

    What part of the patient's body was hurting?

    A. The eye
    B. The ear
    C. The nose
    D. The throat

43. Which suffix would you affix to the word tracheo to complete the following sentence?

    The surgeon needed to perform a tracheo _____ to create an opening in the trachea so the patient could breathe.

    A. -soma
    B. –stat
    C. -scope
    D. -stomy

44. Which of the following words means "treatment with water" for conditions like arthritis or paralysis?

    A. Hydrology
    B. Hydroalgia
    C. Hydropathy
    D. Hydrotherapy

45. Which of the following root words means "sugar"?

    A. Hist
    B. Glyc
    C. Hydr
    D. Kerat

46. In this sentence the root indicates that the patient has inflammation of which body part?

    The patient was suffering from encephalitis.

    A. Liver
    B. Kidney
    C. Spleen
    D. Brain

47. Based on your knowledge of medical roots, prefixes, and suffixes, which of the following words means "the study of the liver, gallbladder, and pancreas"?

    A. Hematology
    B. Hepatology
    C. Gastroenterology
    D. Gynecology

48. Which of the following suffixes means "causing"?

    A. -genic
    B. -tomy
    C. -stasis
    D. -tropic

49. Based on your knowledge of roots, prefixes, and suffixes, what is a neuroplasty?

    A. The damage of a nerve
    B. The inflammation of a nerve
    C. The measurement of a nerve
    D. The surgical repair of a nerve

50. Adding which of the following prefixes to natal would describe the time and events surrounding a birth, or approximately a few weeks before and after it?

    A. Pre-
    B. Epi-
    C. Peri-
    D. Post-

SECTION IV. GRAMMAR

You have 50 minutes to complete 50 questions.

1. **Which of the following spellings is correct?**

   A. Busines
   B. Business
   C. Buseness
   D. Bussiness

2. **Which of the following spellings is correct?**

   A. Argument
   B. Arguemint
   C. Arguement
   D. Arguemant

3. **Which of the following spellings is correct?**

   A. Criticim
   B. Criticism
   C. Kriticism
   D. Critisism

4. **Which of the following spellings is correct?**

   A. Comitment
   B. Comitmant
   C. Comitmment
   D. Commitment

5. **Which word(s) in the following sentence should be capitalized?**

   My friend's birthday is december 25. she does not like that her birthday is on christmas.

   A. christmas
   B. december
   C. december and christmas
   D. december, she, and christmas

6. **Which word(s) in the following sentence should be capitalized?**

   she asked, "do you like indian food?"

   A. she and do
   B. do and indian
   C. she and indian
   D. she, do, and indian

7. **Which word(s) in the following sentence should be capitalized?**

   The three largest cities are new york, los angeles, and chicago.

   A. new, los, and chicago
   B. new york and los angeles
   C. york, angeles, and chicago
   D. new york, los angeles, and chicago

8. **Which word(s) in the following sentence should be capitalized?**

   on wednesdays every other month, the exterminator comes to service the building.

   A. on and wednesdays
   B. on, wednesdays, and month
   C. on, month, and exterminator
   D. wednesdays, month, and exterminator

9. **Which of the following sentences is correct?**

   A. No; I did not do that.
   B. Yes: I ate the leftovers.
   C. No, I am not leaving yet.
   D. Yes I finished my homework.

10. **What is the sentence with the correct use of quotation marks?**

    A. JFK said, Ask not what your country can do for you; ask what you can do for your country.

    B. JFK said, 'Ask not what your country can do for you; ask what you can do for your country.'

    C. JFK said, "Ask not what your country can do for you; ask what you can do for your country."

    D. JFK said a person must not ask what the country can do for them, but what they can do for their country.

11. **What is the sentence with the most correct use of punctuation?**

    A. Wait!   C. Wait-

    B. Wait,   D. Wait;

12. **Which of the following sentences is correct?**

    A. It was good, wasn't it?

    B. Anne did you like the movie?

    C. It had action drama and romance.

    D. Before the movie we went to dinner.

13. **Which of the following words is an abstract noun?**

    A. Car   C. Ruler

    B. Tent   D. Health

14. **Which of the following sentences includes a noun?**

    A. They ran.

    B. We talked it over.

    C. That's easy to fix.

    D. My uncle works hard.

15. **Which proper noun is the subject of the following sentence?**

    Pearl S. Buck is the author of some of my favorite books, including *The Good Earth* and *The Living Reed*.

    A. Reed   C. author

    B. Earth   D. Pearl S. Buck

16. **Which sentence contains a plural noun?**

    A. The child is delightful.

    B. My niece is delightful.

    C. The children are delightful.

    D. My niece and nephew are delightful.

17. **Which word in the following sentence is a possessive pronoun?**

    Are you sure that it's yours?

    A. it's   C. that

    B. you   D. yours

18. **Which pronoun would <u>not</u> work in the following sentence?**

    I asked ____ colleague to bring it to you.

    A. my   C. your

    B. our   D. whose

19. **Which subject correctly completes the following sentence?**

    ____ have tickets to see *Hamilton* next week.

    A. Anybody   C. Sean and me

    B. Sean and I   D. Sean and them

20. Which word in the following sentence is an adjective?

Mrs. Washington loves red roses.

A. Mrs. Washington

B. loves

C. red

D. roses

21. Which word in the following sentence does the underlined adverb describe?

The news is <u>so</u> upsetting.

A. The   C. is

B. news   D. upsetting

22. Which word in the following sentence is an adjective?

That gymnast is so talented.

A. gymnast   C. so

B. is   D. talented

23. Which word in the following sentence is an adjective?

It was a late flight.

A. It   C. late

B. was   D. flight

24. Which word in the following sentence is a conjunction?

Margot can speak English, Russian, and Polish fluently.

A. can   C. and

B. speak   D. fluently

25. Which word is <u>not</u> a preposition?

A. It   C. For

B. At   D. In

26. Which word in the following sentence is an interjection?

"Yikes!" he shouted, as he slipped on the ice.

A. Yikes   C. as

B. shouted   D. on

27. Which word in the following sentence is a preposition?

Our flight will leave at 10:20 a.m.

A. Our   C. at

B. will   D. a.m.

28. What verb tenses are used in the following sentence?

While the burglars were grabbing the money, the police broke down the door.

A. Simple past only

B. Past progressive and simple past

C. Simple past and simple present

D. Present progressive and simple present

29. Which book title contains a verb?

A. *In Our Time*

B. *A Moveable Feast*

C. *The Sun Also Rises*

D. *The Old Man and the Sea*

30. Which sentence does <u>not</u> have a helping verb?

A. They ran.

B. Did they run?

C. They didn't run.

D. Were they running?

25

31. **Select the verb to complete the following sentence.**

    Do you think the automobile or the personal computer ____ changed our lives more?

    A. have
    B. haves
    C. has
    D. his

32. **Select the verb that has the underlined word as its subject in the following sentence.**

    After we add the flour, <u>she</u> wants us to stir the mixture really well.

    A. add
    B. wants
    C. us
    D. stir

33. **Select the word that is <u>not</u> a correct third person singular verb form.**

    A. Does
    B. Its
    C. Wishes
    D. Catches

34. **Select the subject with which the underlined verb must agree.**

    On Memorial Day, which is the last Monday in May, Americans <u>honor</u> those who have died for their country.

    A. Memorial Day
    B. which
    C. Americans
    D. died

35. **Which of the following options would complete the sentence below to make it a compound sentence?**

    The class of middle school students

    _____.

    A. served food at
    B. served food at a soup kitchen
    C. served food at a soup kitchen, and they enjoyed the experience
    D. served food at a soup kitchen even though they weren't required to

36. **Which of the following uses a conjunction to combine the sentences below so the focus is on Tony preparing for his job interview?**

    Tony prepared well for his job interview. Tony ended up getting an offer.

    A. Tony ended up getting an offer; he prepared for his job interview.
    B. Tony prepared well for his job interview, he ended up getting an offer.
    C. Tony prepared well for his job interview and he ended up getting an offer.
    D. Tony ended up getting an offer because he prepared for his job interview.

37. **Which of the following options correctly fixes the run-on sentence below?**

    Texting while driving is reckless it could cost you your life.

    A. Texting while driving is reckless, it could cost you your life.
    B. Texting while driving is reckless it. Could cost you your life.
    C. Texting while driving. Is reckless, it could cost you your life.
    D. Texting while driving is reckless, and it could cost you your life.

38. **Which of the following uses a conjunction to combine the sentences below so the focus is on the people relocating to save money?**

The cost of living is going up in some regions. Many people are relocating to save money.

A. Since the cost of living is going up in some regions, many people are relocating to save money.

B. The cost of living is going up in some regions; many people are relocating to save money.

C. The cost of living is going up in some regions, and many people are relocating to save money.

D. The cost of living is going up in some regions, many people are relocating to save money.

39. **Identify the independent clause in the following sentence.**

After eating dinner, the couple went on a stroll through the park.

A. After eating dinner

B. the couple went on a stroll through the park

C. through the park

D. went on a stroll

40. **Identify the independent clause in the following sentence.**

Although most people understand the benefits of exercise, people do not exercise as much as they should.

A. Although most people understand

B. the benefits of exercise

C. people do not exercise as much as they should

D. people do not exercise

41. **Identify the dependent clause in the following sentence.**

When I lived in New York City, I took the subway to work every day.

A. When I lived in New York City

B. I took the subway

C. to work every day

D. in New York City

42. **Identify the dependent clause in the following sentence.**

While her kids swam in the pool, Nicole read a book.

A. While her kids swam in the pool

B. Nicole read a book

C. swam in the pool

D. While her kids

43. **Which word is a modifier in the following sentence?**

I am following the news story closely.

A. I

B. am

C. following

D. closely

44. Which word in the following sentence is <u>not</u> a modifier?

   That young woman arrived late yesterday.

   A. young   C. late

   B. woman   D. yesterday

45. Which word is a modifier in the following sentence?

   The black dog was barking.

   A. black   C. was

   B. dog   D. barking

46. Which word or phrase does the underlined modifier describe?

   A <u>great</u> time was had by all.

   A. A   C. was had

   B. time   D. by all

47. Select the word that is an object of the underlined verb.

   The graduates <u>held</u> lit candles.

   A. The   C. lit

   B. graduates D. candles

48. Select the verb that acts on the underlined direct object.

   We decided that we should walk <u>the dog</u> before going to the restaurant.

   A. decided   C. walk

   B. should   D. going

49. Select the verb that acts on the underlined direct object in the following sentence.

   We have no choice but to sit here and wait for these cows to cross <u>the road</u>!

   A. have   C. wait

   B. sit   D. cross

50. What part of speech correctly describes the underlined phrase in the following sentence?

   In 1969, man walked on <u>the moon</u>.

   A. Direct object

   B. Indirect object

   C. Object of the preposition

   D. Subject

SECTION V. BIOLOGY

You have 25 minutes to complete 25 questions.

1. In a study, a researcher describes what happens to a plant following exposure to a dry and hot environment. What step of the scientific method does this most likely describe?

   A. Forming a hypothesis

   B. Making an observation

   C. Communicating findings

   D. Characterizing the problem

2. Which is part of the monomer structure of a nucleic acid?

   A. DNA

   B. Glucose

   C. Thymine

   D. Cellulose

3. Which process is anabolic?

   A. Glycolysis

   B. Lipid synthesis

   C. Protein degradation

   D. Oxidative phosphorylation

4. Why are metabolic pathways cyclic?

   A. Metabolic reactions generally take place one at a time.

   B. All of the products created in metabolic reactions are used up.

   C. The reactions are continuous as long as reactants are available.

   D. Energy in the form of ATP is sent to different cells for various uses.

5. Which would benefit from the use of a taxonomic system?

   A. A researcher discovers a new organism while surveying a lake.

   B. A researcher examines the survival of an invasive plant species.

   C. A researcher studies the growth and development of a living thing.

   D. A researcher uses fossils to explain how organisms evolved over time.

6. Why is hydrogen bonding with water important?

   A. It contributes to water's low boiling point.

   B. It prevents water from being a universal solvent.

   C. It creates weak interactions among water molecules.

   D. It allows water in its solid form to float on liquid water.

7. A researcher classifies a newly discovered organism in the class taxonomy level. What other taxonomic level is this new organism classified in?

   A. Order

   B. Family

   C. Species

   D. Kingdom

8. Which statement confirms that the cell membrane is selectively permeable?

   A. Receptors are found on a cell's surface.

   B. Cells communicate with each other using cell signals.

   C. Environmental changes can cause a cell to expand or shrink.

   D. Sodium ions must travel through ion channels to enter the cell.

9. Which organelles work together to protect a plant cell from the external environment?

   A. Flagella and pili

   B. Cytoplasm and lysosome

   C. Cell wall and cell membrane

   D. Ribosome and Golgi apparatus

10. Which organisms are heterotrophs?

   A. Algae   C. Bacteria

   B. Bears   D. Flowers

11. Which organism would most likely be labeled as a consumer?

   A. Archaea   C. Heterotroph

   B. Autotroph   D. Prokaryote

12. Which organelles work together to ensure plant cells have enough energy to use?

   A. Ribosome and nucleus

   B. Chloroplast and mitochondria

   C. Cell membrane and cytoplasm

   D. Golgi apparatus and endoplasmic reticulum

13. Which of the following is supported by the cell theory?

   A. Cells are alive and recognized as the building blocks for life.

   B. Scientists can identify and differentiate cells by using a microscope.

   C. Cells are produced from existing cells using meiosis instead of mitosis.

   D. Living things are composed of a single cell that remains undifferentiated.

14. Why does photosynthesis need ATP?

   A. Make membranes

   B. Establish a gradient

   C. Produce chloroplasts

   D. Create sugar molecules

15. What organism makes a cell plate during cytokinesis?

   A. Bacterium   C. Mushroom

   B. Human   D. Plant

16. Which gives the correct order of cellular respiration?

   A. Glycolysis, Acetyl-CoA, Citric Acid Cycle, Electron Transport Chain

   B. Citric Acid Cycle, Glycolysis, Acetyl-CoA, Electron Transport Chain

   C. Glycolysis, Acetyl-CoA, Electron Transport Chain, Citric Acid Cycle

   D. Glycolysis, Citric Acid Cycle, Electron Transport Chain, Acetyl-CoA

17. What phase is the cell cycle part of?

   A. Interphase   C. Prophase

   B. Metaphase   D. Telophase

18. What metabolic process helps a cell yield a large amount of ATP?

   A. Glycolysis

   B. Chemiosmosis

   C. Citric acid cycle

   D. Oxidation of pyruvate

19. A child falls down and punctures his skin. What biological process must occur to repair the damaged skin?

   A. Glycolysis

   B. Cell respiration

   C. Gluconeogenesis

   D. Cell reproduction

20. What is the function of a peptide bond?

   A. To connect proteins together

   B. To connect nucleotides together

   C. To connect amino acids together

   D. To connect nucleic acids together

21. What is the end product of translation?

   A. Amino acids

   B. Stop codons

   C. Transfer RNA

   D. Messenger RNA

22. What is the purpose of RNA polymerase?

   A. To become a protein

   B. To become a nucleotide

   C. To function as an enzyme

   D. To develop into a terminator

23. Right before cell division, a DNA molecule and its associated proteins

   A. coil tightly.

   B. stretch out.

   C. form a double helix.

   D. wrap around each other.

24. What is the function of a centromere?

   A. To connect the two chromatids

   B. To keep the chromosome stable

   C. To act as a relay point for genetic information

   D. To transmit genetic codes between other chromosomes

25. Mendel discovered the pattern associated with _____ after developing a series of rules in genetics.

   A. epigenetics

   B. heredity

   C. heterogeneity

   D. taxonomy

SECTION VI. CHEMISTRY

You have 25 minutes to complete 25 questions.

1. An electric balance measures an object's

    A. mass.

    B. length.

    C. temperature.

    D. volume.

2. Several participants are enrolled in a study that is evaluating the effectiveness of new drug targeted at slowing the progression of breast cancer. Some participants are asked to take the new drug and monitored over a six-month period. Others are asked to take a placebo. They are also monitored over six months. What is the dependent variable?

    A. Drug

    B. Condition

    C. Placebo

    D. Time

3. Five tropical plants are kept at varying humidity levels in a greenhouse for three months. One plant is left outside in normal conditions. Plant height is measured weekly. What is the control of the experiment?

    A. Plant height for each tropical plant

    B. The plant left outside in normal conditions

    C. Humidity level readings in the greenhouse

    D. Amount of time used to study plant height

4. Deductive reasoning is a logical process based on

    A. working with data to formulate a hypothesis.

    B. drawing conclusions from a specific observation.

    C. using a general idea to make a specific conclusion.

    D. relying on empirical evidence to answer questions.

5. Atom X has an atomic number of 10 and a mass of 20 amu. Atom Y has 10 protons and 12 neutrons. Which of the following describes the relationship between these atoms?

    A. They are different elements.

    B. They are isotopes of the same element.

    C. They have the same atomic number and the same atomic mass.

    D. They have different atomic numbers and different atomic masses.

6. Which of the following describes a neutral atom of tin-120?

    A. 50 protons, 70 neutrons, 50 electrons

    B. 50 protons, 120 neutrons, 50 electrons

    C. 50 protons, 120 neutrons, 70 electrons

    D. 70 protons, 120 neutrons, 70 electrons

7. How many electrons does a neutral atom of iodine have?

    A. 53

    B. 74

    C. 126

    D. 127

8. An atom has 28 protons, 32 neutrons, and 28 electrons. What is the name of this isotope?

   A. Nickel-32
   B. Nickel-60
   C. Germanium-56
   D. Germanium-60

9. How many kilograms are in 1,800 grams?

   A. 0.18   C. 18
   B. 1.8   D. 180

10. How many cups are in 22 pints?

   A. 11   C. 24
   B. 20   D. 44

11. How many inches are in 35 centimeters?

   A. 0.035   C. 31.85
   B. 13.77   D. 88.90

12. One centigram of a substance is equal to how many grams?

   A. 0.0001   C. 10
   B. 0.01   D. 1000

13. At the end of which phase change will a substance have less energy than it did at the beginning?

   A. Deposition   C. Sublimation
   B. Melting   D. Vaporization

14. A substance will _____ at the same temperature.

   A. melt and boil
   B. condense and boil
   C. freeze and sublime
   D. freeze and condense

15. As a substance _____, the particles in the substance get closer together.

   A. boils   C. melts
   B. condenses   D. sublimes

16. What is the difference between evaporation and boiling?

   A. Evaporation occurs throughout a substance, and boiling occurs on the bottom of it.
   B. Evaporation occurs on the surface of a substance, and boiling occurs throughout it.
   C. Evaporation occurs on the bottom of a substance, and boiling occurs on the surface of it.
   D. Evaporation occurs on the surface of a substance, and boiling occurs on the bottom of it.

17. The amount of heat that has been removed from the substance allows the particles to draw closer together, and the material changes from a liquid to a solid. Which of the following is being described?

   A. Condensation   C. Freezing
   B. Deposition   D. Sublimation

18. A neutral atom has two electrons in its first energy shell, eight electrons in its second energy shell, and three electrons in its third energy shell. Which electrons will be lost when the atom reacts to become stable?

   A. Electrons in the first shell
   B. Electrons in the second shell
   C. Electrons in the third shell
   D. Electrons in the second or third shell

19. How many potassium and nitrogen ions are needed to form an ionic compound?

    A. One potassium ion and one nitrogen ion

    B. Three potassium ions and one nitrogen ion

    C. One potassium ion and three nitrogen ions

    D. Three potassium ions and three nitrogen ions

20. What is the net charge of the ionic compound barium iodide (BaI_2)?

    A. -1   C. +1

    B. 0   D. +2

21. What type of reaction is described by the following equation?

    $2Na(s) + ZnCl_2(aq)$ $Zn(s) + 2NaCl(aq)$

    A. Synthesis

    B. Combustion

    C. Single-replacement

    D. Double-replacement

22. In which reaction do the reactants form a homogeneous mixture and the products form a heterogeneous mixture?

    A. $CaO(s) + H_2O(l)$ $Ca(OH)_2(s)$

    B. $C_3H_8(g) + 5O_2(g)$ $3CO_2(g) + 4H_2O(g)$

    C. $2Na(s) + ZnCl_2(aq)$ $Zn(s) + 2NaCl(aq)$

    D. $Pb(NO_3)_2(aq) + 2KI(aq)$ $PbI_2(s) + 2KNO_3(aq)$

23. What is the conjugate base in the following reaction?

    $HNO_2 + H_2O \longleftrightarrow$?

    A. OH^- C. H_3O^+

    B. NO_2^- D. HNO_3^-

24. When HNO_3 reacts with NaOH, which product is formed?

    A. OH^- C. NaH

    B. H_3O^+ D. $NaNO_3$

25. Which of the following is a strong acid?

    A. HF   C. H_3PO_4

    B. HCl   D. CH_3COOH

SECTION VII. ANATOMY & PHYSIOLOGY

You have 25 minutes to complete 25 questions.

1. Which plane of the body divides the body into two equal halves?

   A. Coronal   C. Sagittal

   B. Midsagittal   D. Transverse

2. _____ is a point in the functioning of a human body where everything is working optimally.

   A. Diffusion   C. Metabolism

   B. Homeostasis   D. Variable

3. What substances transported in blood does the liver excrete as bile?

   A. Gases   C. Nutrients

   B. Hormones   D. Wastes

4. After blood leaves the aorta, it travels to the

   A. arteries.   C. capillaries.

   B. arterioles.   D. venules.

5. Why is it important to secrete mucous from epithelial cells?

   A. It helps the diaphragm change shape.

   B. It increases the surface area of the alveoli.

   C. It lubricates the lungs for easier movement.

   D. It prevents particles from entering the lungs.

6. A characteristic of alveoli is that they are

   A. attached to the bronchi.

   B. connected to the diaphragm.

   C. known to have a small surface area.

   D. tiny air sacs where gas exchange occurs.

7. The cardiac sphincter opens into the _____.

   A. gallbladder   C. pancreas

   B. liver   D. stomach

8. Which of the following molecules is able to diffuse through the lining of the small intestine?

   A. Glycerol   C. Polypeptides

   B. Peptides   D. Sucrose

9. The female reproductive system includes _____.

   A. uterus and cervix

   B. epididymis and Fallopian tube

   C. ovaries, prostate gland, and vagina

   D. ovaries, uterus, and corpus cavernosum

10. Humans utilize which type of reproduction?

    A. Binary fission

    B. Parthenogenesis

    C. Sexual reproduction

    D. Asexual reproduction

11. Which structure is part of the renal tubule?

    A. Urethra

    B. Glomerulus

    C. Collecting duct

    D. Bowman's capsule

12. Which describes one function of the urinary system?

    A. Reabsorb nitrogenous wastes

    B. Osmoregulate blood and water

    C. Push urine out of the body via the ureter

    D. Secrete hormones from endocrine glands

13. At which of the following ages would ossification most likely take place to replace cartilage at the growth plate?

    A. 5   C. 42

    B. 18   D. 91

14. What is a benefit of bone resorption?

    A. Releasing minerals into blood circulation

    B. Transforming soft tissue to hard connective tissue

    C. Creating avenues for nerve fibers to travel in bone

    D. Stimulating hematopoiesis for red blood cell development

15. Which describes the shape of a skeletal muscle cell?

    A. Branched   C. Short

    B. Elongated   D. Spindle

16. Which structure cushions bones at the point where they meet?

    A. Joint   C. Ligament

    B. Tendon   D. Sarcomere

17. When a flexor muscles contracts, an extension muscle _____.

    A. elongates   C. recoils

    B. pivots   D. shortens

18. A person jumps after touching a hot surface. Which layer of skin was responsible for stimulating the person's response?

    A. Dermis

    B. Hypodermis

    C. Stratum basale

    D. Stratum lucidum

19. The epidermis is made of _____ layers.

    A. 2   C. 5

    B. 3   D. 8

20. What is a major structure of the limbic system?

    A. Brainstem

    B. Spinal cord

    C. Hypothalamus

    D. Cerebral cortex

21. What sense bypasses the thalamus as the CNS processes sensory information?

    A. Hearing   C. Smelling

    B. Seeing   D. Touching

22. Which of the following could be a result of the effects of aging on hormones?

    A. Poor sight

    B. Loss of strength

    C. Change in moods

    D. Fluctuating weight

23. The thyroid-stimulating hormone's response is an increased metabolic rate. What would be a side effect of an underactive secretion rate?

    A. Hot flashes

    B. Weight gain

    C. Mood swings

    D. Increased energy

24. HIV/AIDS disables the immune system by _____.

    A. blocking the action of T cells

    B. triggering genetic mutations

    C. activating the production of B cells

    D. destroying helper T cells and macrophages

25. Rheumatoid arthritis attacks on membranes around the joints are an example of a(n) _____.

    A. immunity

    B. pathogen

    C. allergic response

    D. autoimmune disease

SECTION VIII. PHYSICS

You have 50 minutes to complete 25 questions.

1. Which process could serve as a way to consistently measure time?

    A. The growth of a tree

    B. The phases of the moon

    C. The chirping of a cricket

    D. The water height of a river

2. A 2.0-kilogram object experiences a net force of 144 newtons. What is its acceleration?

    A. 36 m/s²

    B. 72 m/s²

    C. 140 m/s²

    D. 290 m/s²

3. A 3.0-kilogram object moving northward experiences a southward force of 75 newtons. What is its acceleration?

    A. 25 m/s² northward

    B. 25 m/s² southward

    C. 225 m/s² northward

    D. 225 m/s² southward

4. Given any two vectors $\vec{a}$ and $\vec{b}$ and any scalar c, which expression is always true?

    A. $c\vec{a} = c\vec{b}$

    B. $\vec{a} + \vec{b} = c$

    C. $\vec{a} - \vec{b} = \vec{b} - \vec{a}$

    D. $\vec{a} + \vec{b} = \vec{b} + \vec{a}$

5. An object is moving with a velocity (−2.12, 6.37) in meters per second. What is its speed?

    A. 2.91 m/s

    B. 4.25 m/s

    C. 6.01 m/s

    D. 6.72 m/s

6. A merry-go-round is spinning counterclockwise. If a child riding the merry-go-round jumps off when he is experiencing centripetal acceleration directed southward, in what direction will he be moving when he hits the ground?

    A. East

    B. North

    C. South

    D. West

7. A student conducting a physics experiment drives a car with a blindfolded passenger and asks that passenger to determine whether the car's motion is linear or nonlinear. Which experience tells the passenger that the car is moving nonlinearly?

    A. The passenger feels no forces.

    B. The passenger feels a constant backward force.

    C. The passenger feels an increasing forward force.

    D. The passenger feels a decreasing sideways force.

8. A racecar moving clockwise on a circular track is subject to friction from air resistance and contact between the tires and the track. If the driver is to maintain uniform circular motion, what must he do?

    A. Hit the brake

    B. Hit the gas pedal

    C. Turn the wheel farther to the left

    D. Turn the wheel farther to the right

9. A plane is flying at a constant speed on a circular path as the pilots wait for permission to land. If a 65-kilogram passenger feels a centrifugal force of 25 newtons, what is the plane's centripetal acceleration?

   A. 0.38 m/s²

   B. 0.76 m/s²

   C. 2.6 m/s²

   D. 1,600 m/s²

10. Which parameter of uniform circular motion can vary independently of the other three?

    A. Period

    B. Frequency

    C. Angular frequency

    D. Centripetal acceleration

11. Materials X and Y have the same compressibility, but X is denser than Y. Which statement is correct?

    A. Sound waves will travel in X but not in Y.

    B. Sound waves will travel faster in X than in Y.

    C. Sound waves will travel faster in Y than in X.

    D. Sound waves will travel at the same speed in X and Y.

12. Which of the following best describes an atom's nucleus?

    A. A tightly packed combination of neutrons and protons

    B. A tightly packed combination of electrons and protons

    C. A tightly packed combination of electrons and neutrons

    D. A tightly packed combination of electrons, neutrons, and protons

13. Which situation falls in the domain of optics?

    A. Magnification of an object by a lens

    B. Propagation of sound through a solid material

    C. Diffraction of ocean waves at the entrance to a cove

    D. Refraction of seismic waves caused by an earthquake

14. Two parallel mirrors are facing each other. If a light ray strikes one mirror at a 0° angle from the normal, at what angle will it reflect from the other mirror?

    A. 0° from the normal

    B. 45° from the normal

    C. 60° from the normal

    D. 90° from the normal

15. If a sound wave in air at a certain temperature and humidity has a frequency of 125 Hz and a wavelength of 9.00 feet, what is its wave speed?

    A. 0.0720 feet per second

    B. 13.9 feet per second

    C. 134 feet per second

    D. 1,125 feet per second

16. What is the gravitational attraction force between the space shuttle (2,031,000 kg) and the Hubble Space Telescope (11,110 kg) when they are 50.0 m apart?

    A. 6.02×10^{-4} N

    B. 6.02 N

    C. 60.2 N

    D. 6.02×10^{4} N

17. A freight car has a momentum of $300,000 \frac{kg \cdot m}{s}$ while moving along a frictionless, level railroad track with a constant speed of 15 m/s. What is the mass of the freight car in kg?

   A. 1,000

   B. 2,000

   C. 20,000

   D. 200,000

18. What is the mass, in grams, of an arrow shot at 101 m/s if a bale of hay imparts 12 N of force during the 0.20 s it takes to halt the arrow?

   A. 12

   B. 24

   C. 36

   D. 48

19. What is the height above ground of a 55 g egg that possesses 0.27 J of potential energy?

   A. 0.00050 m

   B. 0.0050 m

   C. 0.050 m

   D. 0.50 m

20. What is the momentum of a golf ball with a mass of 45.9 g moving at 81 m/s in $\frac{kg \cdot m}{s}$?

   A. 1.4

   B. 2.0

   C. 3.3

   D. 3.7

21. Which of the following represents an electric current?

   A. Electric flux in a vacuum

   B. Electrons moving in a wire

   C. A disconnected voltage source

   D. An electromagnetic wave in a material

22. A circuit contains a battery and a 2-ohm resistor. If 0.001 amps of current flow from the battery's positive terminal, how much current flows back into its negative terminal?

   A. 0 amps

   B. 0.0005 amps

   C. 0.001 amps

   D. 0.002 amps

23. What is the electric field precisely halfway between two 0.001-coulomb charges spaced 1 meter apart? (Assume the electric constant is 9×10^9 when using units of newtons, coulombs, and meters.)

   A. 0 newtons per coulomb

   B. 9,000 newtons per coulomb

   C. 9,000,000 newtons per coulomb

   D. 9,000,000,000 newtons per coulomb

24. A 5.0-volt battery delivers 0.020 amps to a resistor. What is the resistance of the resistor?

   A. 4.0×10^{-3} ohms

   B. 0.10 ohms

   C. 10 ohms

   D. 250 ohms

25. A 100-ohm resistor has a current of 0.01 amps flowing through it. What is the voltage across the resistor?

   A. 0.01 volts

   B. 1 volt

   C. 100 volts

   D. 10,000 volts

HESI PRACTICE EXAM 1
ANSWER KEY WITH EXPLANATORY ANSWERS

Section I. Mathematics

1. **B.** The correct solution is the whole numbers include zero, but the natural numbers exclude zero. The natural or "counting" numbers are 1, 2, 3, 4,.... To get the whole numbers, just include 0 with the natural numbers. **Skill: Basic Addition and Subtraction.**

2. **A.** The correct solution is 1,078. Adding any number to 0 yields that number. On a number line, starting at a certain number and taking no steps in either direction yields the same number. **Skill: Basic Addition and Subtraction.**

3. **C.** The correct solution is 3,047. Place the digits in base-10 format, using the number of meters in the thousands place, the number of centimeters in the tens place, and the number of millimeters in the ones place. The measurement is 3,047 millimeters long. **Skill: Basic Addition and Subtraction.**

4. **B.** The correct solution is −19. Because the subtraction algorithm does not apply directly in this case (the first number is smaller than the second), first use the rule that $x - y = -(y - x)$. So, $8 - 27 = -(27 - 8)$. Applying the algorithm to $27 - 8$ yields 19, then $-(27 - 8) = -19$. **Skill: Basic Addition and Subtraction.**

5. **A.** The correct solution is −10, 0, 1, 8. One approach is to place the numbers on the number line and make sure they appear from left to right in the same order they appear in the answers above. Alternatively, note that negative numbers are less than positive numbers (and 0), then order the remaining numbers. **Skill: Basic Addition and Subtraction.**

6. **D.** When dividing whole numbers, the remainder is the portion of the dividend left over after finding the whole-number part of the quotient. The remainder is always smaller than the divisor. **Skill: Basic Multiplication and Division.**

7. **A.** Use the division algorithm. Knowing the multiplication table well helps you recognize these numbers. **Skill: Basic Multiplication and Division.**

8. **C.** Carefully follow the order of operations. First, multiply and divide from left to right. Then, add. **Skill: Basic Multiplication and Division.**

$12 \div 4 \times 3 + 1$

$3 \times 3 + 1$

$9 + 1$

10

9. C. Use the multiplication algorithm. It involves adding 84 and 1,120 to get the product of 1,204. **Skill: Basic Multiplication and Division.**

10. B. One of the two basic rules for multiplying signed numbers is that if the numbers have the same sign, their product is positive. **Skill: Basic Multiplication and Division.**

11. B. The correct solution is $\frac{7}{11}$. Let $n = 0.\overline{63}$ and $100n = 63.\overline{63}$ Then, $100n-n = 63.\overline{63}-0.\overline{63}$ resulting in $99n = 63$ and solution of $n = \frac{63}{99} = \frac{7}{11}$. **Skill: Decimals and Fractions.**

12. A. The correct solution is $\frac{5}{12}$ because $\frac{5}{12}$ has the largest numerator when comparing to the other fractions with the same denominator. The fractions with a common denominator of 12 are $\frac{5}{12} = \frac{5}{12}, \frac{1}{3} = \frac{4}{12}, \frac{1}{6} = \frac{2}{12}, \frac{1}{4} = \frac{3}{12}$. **Skill: Decimals and Fractions.**

13. C. The correct solution is 4.44 because 4.44 contains the largest values in the tenths and hundredths places. **Skill: Decimals and Fractions.**

14. C. The correct solution is 0.687 because 0.687 contains the smallest value in the tenths place. **Skill: Decimals and Fractions.**

15. C. The correct solution is $\frac{8}{45}$ because $\frac{2}{3} \times \frac{4}{15} = \frac{8}{45}$. **Skill: Multiplication and Division of Fractions.**

16. A. The correct solution is $\frac{3}{28}$ because $\frac{3}{16} \times \frac{4}{7} = \frac{12}{112} = \frac{3}{28}$. **Skill: Multiplication and Division of Fractions.**

17. C. The correct solution is $\frac{3}{20}$ because $\frac{1}{10} \times \frac{3}{2} = \frac{3}{20}$. **Skill: Multiplication and Division of Fractions.**

18. C. The correct solution is $1\frac{11}{45}$ because $\frac{8}{9} \times \frac{7}{5} = \frac{56}{45} = 1\frac{11}{45}$. **Skill: Multiplication and Division of Fractions.**

19. D. The correct answer is D. Although solving each proportion is one approach, the easiest approach is to compare them as they are. The proportions in answers A and B yield the same number for the unknown because they keep the same numbers in either the numerators or the denominators. Answer C just reverses the order of the equation in answer A, which does not yield a different number for the unknown. Answer D flips one fraction without flipping the other, which changes the proportion. **Skill: Ratios, Proportions, and Percentages.**

20. C. There are 300 cattle in the herd. Because the herd is only Ayrshire or Jersey, it is 65% Jersey. The equivalent decimals are 0.35 Ayrshire and 0.65 Jersey. Set up a proportion that relates these decimals to the number of cattle of each type:

$$\frac{0.35}{0.65} = \frac{?}{195}$$

One approach is to divide 195 by 0.65 to get 300, then multiply by 0.35 to get the number of Ayrshires: 105. Add 195 and 105 to get the total number of cattle in the herd. **Skill: Ratios, Proportions, and Percentages.**

21. B. The number 147 satisfies the proportion. First, divide 378 by 18 to get 21. Then, multiply 21 by 7 to get 147. Check your answer by dividing 147 by 7: the quotient is also 21, so 147 satisfies the proportion. **Skill: Ratios, Proportions, and Percentages.**

22. B. First, convert the fraction $\frac{15}{250}$ to a decimal: 0.06. To get the percent, multiply by 100% (that is, multiply by 100 and add the % symbol). Of all entries, 6% are winners. **Skill: Ratios, Proportions, and Percentages.**

23. C. The ratio 4:5 is equal to $\frac{4}{5}$, or 0.8. Multiply by 100% to get 80%. **Skill: Ratios, Proportions, and Percentages.**

24. D. The correct solution is 13,200 feet. $2.5 \text{ mi} \times \frac{5280 \text{ ft}}{1 \text{ mi}} = 13,200 \text{ ft}$. **Skill: Standards of Measure.**

25. A. The correct solution is 0.147 kiloliters. $147 \text{ L} \times \frac{1 \text{ kL}}{1,000 \text{ L}} = \frac{147}{1,000} = 0.147 \text{ kL}$. **Skill: Standards of Measure.**

26. A. The correct solution is $1\frac{1}{3}$ yards. $48 \text{ in} \times \frac{1 \text{ ft}}{12 \text{ in}} \times \frac{1 \text{ yd}}{3 \text{ ft}} = \frac{48}{36} = 1\frac{1}{3} \text{ yd}$. **Skill: Standards of Measure.**

27. C. The correct solution is 18,000 millimeters. $18 \, m \times \frac{1,000 \, mm}{1 \, m} = 18,000 \, mm$. **Skill: Standards of Measure.**

28. D. The correct solution is 2:35 p.m. Subtract 1200 from the time, $1435 - 1200 = 2:35$ p.m. **Skill: Standards of Measure.**

29. D. The correct solution is 48 because both sides of the equation are multiplied by −4. **Skill: Equations with One Variable.**

30. D. The correct solution is $x \geq 3$.

$3x + 3 + 2x + 2 \geq 15 - 5x + 4x + 8$	Apply the distributive property.
$5x + 5 \geq -x + 23$	Combine like terms on both sides of the inequality.
$6x + 5 \geq 23$	Add x to both sides of the inequality.
$6x \geq 18$	Subtract 5 from both sides of the inequality.
$x \geq 3$	Divide both sides of the inequality by 6.

Skill: Equations with One Variable.

31. D. The correct solution is $x \geq \frac{1}{15}$.

$3x-4(x+2) \leq 2x+3+12x-12$	Multiply all terms by the least common denominator of 12 to eliminate the fractions.
$3x-4x-8 \leq 2x+3+12x-12$	Apply the distributive property.
$-x-8 \leq 14x-9$	Combine like terms on both sides of the inequality.
$-15x-8 \leq -9$	Subtract $14x$ from both sides of the inequality.
$-15x \leq -1$	Add 8 to both sides of the inequality.
$x \geq \frac{1}{15}$	Divide both sides of the inequality by -15.

Skill: Equations with One Variable.

32. B. The correct solution is -6 because both sides of the equation are divided by -6. **Skill: Equations with One Variable.**

33. C. The correct solution is (1, 3).

	The first equation is already solved for x.
$-3y+10 = 3y-8$	Substitute $-3y+10$ in for x in the second equation.
$-6y+10 = -8$	Subtract $3y$ from both sides of the equation.
$-6y = -18$	Subtract 10 from both sides of the equation.
$y = 3$	Divide both sides of the equation by -6.
$x = -3(3)+10$	Substitute 3 in the first equation for y.
$x = -9+10 = 1$	Simplify using order of operations.

Skill: Equations with Two Variables.

34. A. The correct solution is (0, -4).

	The first equation is already solved for y.
$-4x-4 = -5x-4$	Substitute $-4x-4$ in for y in the second equation.
$x-4 = -4$	Add $5x$ to both sides of the equation.
$x = 0$	Add 4 to both sides of the equation.
$y = -4(0)-4$	Substitute 0 in the first equation for x.
$y = 0-4 = -4$	Simplify using order of operations.

Skill: Equations with Two Variables.

35. B. The correct solution is (-10, 3).

	The first equation is already solved for x.
$-(-y-7) + 4y = 22$	Substitute $-y-7$ in for x in the second equation.
$y + 7 + 4y = 22$	Apply the distributive property.
$5y + 7 = 22$	Combine like terms on the left side of the equation.
$5y = 15$	Subtract 7 from both sides of the equation.
$y = 3$	Divide both sides of the equation by 5.
$x = -3-7$	Substitute 3 in the first equation for y.
$x = -10$	Simplify using order of operations.

Skill: Equations with Two Variables.

36. A. The correct solution is -520 because $-8 \times 65 = -520$ points. **Skill: Solving Real World Mathematical Problems.**

37. B. The correct solution is -1 because the sum of the scores is -10. The average is -10 divided by 10, or -1 point. **Skill: Solving Real World Mathematical Problems.**

38. C. The correct solution is 1,530 because $1,450-(-80) = 1,450 + 80 = 1,530$ feet. **Skill: Solving Real World Mathematical Problems.**

39. B. The correct solution is $900 because $-300 + (-300) + (-100) + 400 + 600 + 600 = \$900$. **Skill: Solving Real World Mathematical Problems.**

40. D. The correct solution is 15 because the first athlete's salary is about \$30,000,000 and the second athlete's salary is about \$2,000,000. So, the first athlete's salary is about 15 times larger. **Skill: Powers, Exponents, Roots, and Radicals.**

41. D. The correct solution is $16x^6$ because $(4x^3)^2 = 4^2 x^{3 \times 2} = 4^2 x^6 = 16x^6$. **Skill: Powers, Exponents, Roots, and Radicals.**

42. C. The correct graph has the two lines intersect at (-9, -1). **Skill: Equations with Two Variables.**

43. C. The correct solution is $-15, 15$ because the square root of 225 is 15. The values of -15 and 15 make the equation true. **Skill: Powers, Exponents, Roots, and Radicals.**

44. A. The correct solution is $\frac{1}{216}$ because $(6^3)^{-1} = 6^{3 \times (-1)} = 6^{-3} = \frac{1}{6^3} = \frac{1}{216}$. **Skill: Powers, Exponents, Roots, and Radicals.**

45. D. The correct solution is $-9, 9$ because the square root of 81 is 9. The values of -9 and 9 make the equation true. **Skill: Powers, Exponents, Roots, and Radicals.**

46. A. The correct solution is $(x + 5)(x^2-5x + 25)$. The expression $x^3 + 125$ is rewritten as $(x + 5)(x^2-5x + 25)$ because the value of a is x and the value of b is 5. **Skill: Polynomials.**

47. A. The correct solution is $-6x^2y^2 + 2x^3y^3$.

$$2xy(-3xy + x^2y^2) = 2xy(-3xy) + 2xy(x^2y^2) = -6x^2y^2 + 2x^3y^3$$

Skill: Polynomials.

48. D. The correct graph has the two lines intersect at (0, 3). **Skill: Equations with Two Variables.**

49. B. The correct solution is $(x + 10)^2$. The expression $x^2 + 20x + 100$ is rewritten as $(x + 10)^2$ because the value of a is x and the value of b is 10. **Skill: Polynomials.**

50. C. The correct solution is $2x^2 + 5xy - 11y^2$.

$(6x^2 + 3xy - 5y^2) - (4x^2 - 2xy + 6y^2) = (6x^2 + 3xy - 5y^2) + (-4x^2 + 2xy - 6y^2) = (6x^2 - 4x^2) + (3xy + 2xy) + (-5y^2 - 6y^2) = 2x^2 + 5xy - 11y^2$

Skill: Polynomials.

Section II. Reading Comprehension

1. B. The second sentence of this paragraph expresses the main idea that chocolate chip cookies were invented by accident. This makes it the topic sentence. **Skill: Main Ideas, Topic Sentences, and Supporting Details.**

2. A. The topic of a sentence is a word or phrase that describes what the text is about. **Skill: Main Ideas, Topic Sentences, and Supporting Details.**

3. C. This paragraph presents the story behind the invention of the chocolate chip cookie. It discusses the fact that the dessert was a complete accident. This idea is expressed in a topic sentence at the beginning of the paragraph. **Skill: Main Ideas, Topic Sentences, and Supporting Details.**

4. D. The main idea of this paragraph is that chocolate chip cookies were invented by accident. The detail that directly supports this is the one describing what Ruth Graves Wakefield did when she ran out of baker's chocolate – she broke up a block of Nestle semi-sweet chocolate expecting them to melt. This is a supporting detail. **Skill: Main Ideas, Topic Sentences, and Supporting Details.**

5. B. All of the above sentences relate to the topic of chocolate chip cookies, but only the sentence about Ruth Graves Wakefield realizing how delicious they were relates directly to the main idea that the chocolate chip cookie was invented by accident. **Skill: Main Ideas, Topic Sentences, and Supporting Details.**

6. B. All of the above sentences are related in some way to the text, but the topic is specifically about an account of human impact on an animal species. **Skill: Main Ideas, Topic Sentences, and Supporting Details.**

7. C. The best topic sentence to unite the above information would be the one about human encroachment negatively impacting the koala population. The others would be additional supporting details. **Skill: Main Ideas, Topic Sentences, and Supporting Details.**

8. D. Each of the above sentences is related in some way to the passage, but the detail about the number of koala pathways that have been built is the best fit for the topic of the text. **Skill: Main Ideas, Topic Sentences, and Supporting Details.**

9. A. A diagram presents a picture with labels that show the parts of an object or functions of a mechanism. This would be the best graphic to support the paragraph mentioned above. **Skill: Summarizing Text and Using Text Features.**

10. D. A pie chart is useful for representing all of something – in this case a large donation made to a charity – and the percentage values of its parts. **Skill: Summarizing Text and Using Text Features.**

11. B. This summary is effective because it restates only the key points and it does it using new words. **Skill: Summarizing Text and Using Text Features.**

12. A. An ineffective summary would copy the original text word for word and only change one or two words. The first sentence is almost exactly like the first sentence of the original text, so this would be structurally plagiarized. **Skill: Summarizing Text and Using Text Features.**

13. B. The words "Then" and "Next" indicate sequence because they tell you when to do a step. **Skill: Summarizing Text and Using Text Features.**

14. B. The prefix "pre" in the word "pre-greased" means "before," so the cookie sheet needs to be greased sometime before putting the batter onto it. **Skill: Summarizing Text and Using Text Features.**

15. B. Since this is the final step, you would use the word "last" to indicate it is the final step in the directions. **Skill: Summarizing Text and Using Text Features.**

16. D. The sentences would be best served with an example transition and an addition transition. **Skill: Tone, Mood, and Transition Words.**

17. A. Transition words like "however" express a contrast between ideas. **Skill: Tone, Mood, and Transition Words.**

18. C. The transition is the word that links the two ideas: *thus*. This word shows how the two sentences have a cause-and-effect relationship. **Skill: Tone, Mood, and Transition Words.**

19. C. The transition is the word that links the two ideas: *also*. The word *however* here is not a transition word indicating contrast; it's an adverb meaning "in whichever way." **Skill: Tone, Mood, and Transition Words.**

20. D. The tone of this letter is appreciative as the author openly thanks the teacher for all he has done for her daughter. **Skill: Tone, Mood, and Transition Words.**

21. D. The author of the letter uses a lot of respectful and admiring language, but the line "We cannot thank you enough" has an especially appreciative and warm tone. **Skill: Tone, Mood, and Transition Words.**

22. B. A teacher receiving a note like this would likely feel grateful. **Skill: Tone, Mood, and Transition Words.**

23. D. The phrase "above all" adds emphasis to the writer's point that the teacher has made a significant impact on the daughter. **Skill: Tone, Mood, and Transition Words.**

24. B. An author's purpose is his or her reason for writing. **Skill: Understanding Author's Purpose, Point of View, and Rhetorical Strategies.**

25. B. Informational texts like cookbooks are usually meant to inform. **Skill: Understanding Author's Purpose, Point of View, and Rhetorical Strategies.**

26. C. The article argues a point, so it is meant to persuade. **Skill: Understanding Author's Purpose, Point of View, and Rhetorical Strategies.**

27. D. Entertaining texts tell stories. This story is about one family's experience moving to a foreign country. **Skill: Understanding Author's Purpose, Point of View, and Rhetorical Strategies.**

28. C. Passage 1 is intended to persuade readers that termites are amazing insects. **Skill: Understanding Author's Purpose, Point of View, and Rhetorical Strategies.**

29. D. Passage 2 tells a story, which is meant to entertain. **Skill: Understanding Author's Purpose, Point of View, and Rhetorical Strategies.**

30. A. Passage 1 says, "Many people find termites to be destructive little pests, but they are actually ingenious little creatures." This suggests that termites are misunderstood and things are not always what they seem. **Skill: Understanding Author's Purpose, Point of View, and Rhetorical Strategies.**

31. B. The author of Passage 1 uses primarily facts and logic, although she could strengthen her points by clearly identifying sources or establishing her credentials. **Skill: Understanding Author's Purpose, Point of View, and Rhetorical Strategies.**

32. A. The argument that getting rid of homework is undoubtedly beneficial is an opinion statement because it makes a judgment. **Skill: Facts, Opinions, and Evaluating an Argument.**

33. C. The statement is a fact because it discusses the results of standardized test scores, which can be measured. **Skill: Facts, Opinions, and Evaluating an Argument.**

34. B. The main argument in this passage is that there are no clear benefits from giving elementary aged students daily homework. **Skill: Facts, Opinions, and Evaluating an Argument.**

35. D. The sentence about homework doing nothing to enhance student learning at all is an overgeneralization. The term "at all" makes a big over-arching claim that cannot be verified, as the author does not even explore some of the potential benefits of daily homework. **Skill: Facts, Opinions, and Evaluating an Argument.**

36. B. This passage argues that childhood obesity is a major problem in our country. **Skill: Facts, Opinions, and Evaluating an Argument.**

37. B. Factual information is verifiable and not based on personal beliefs or feelings. The statistic about the number of children who have been diagnosed as obese is a fact. **Skill: Facts, Opinions, and Evaluating an Argument.**

38. A. This statement takes a complex issue and presents it as if only two possible options are in play. This is an either/or fallacy. **Skill: Facts, Opinions, and Evaluating an Argument.**

39. C. The sentence in question is an example of circular reasoning. That is, it restates the argument in different words instead of providing evidence to back it up. **Skill: Facts, Opinions, and Evaluating an Argument.**

40. A. The phrase "very overweight" in this sentence reflects a judgment that is subject to interpretation. This indicates that the sentence reflects a belief rather than a fact. **Skill: Facts, Opinions, and Evaluating an Argument.**

41. D. Primary sources are written by people who witnessed the original creation or discovery of the information they present. An interview would be an example of a primary source. **Skill: Understanding Primary Sources, Making Inferences, and Drawing Conclusions.**

42. B. Secondary sources respond to, analyze, summarize, or comment on primary sources. In this case, the artist's work is considered the primary source, so the commentary on the artwork would be a secondary source. **Skill: Understanding Primary Sources, Making Inferences, and Drawing Conclusions.**

43. A. Readers must use judgment to determine how credible a source is in a particular circumstance. An op-ed piece in a newspaper would be biased since it expresses the opinion of the author. **Skill: Understanding Primary Sources, Making Inferences, and Drawing Conclusions.**

44. D. An article about Betty Friedan's contributions to the women's movement would be a secondary source. **Skill: Understanding Primary Sources, Making Inferences, and Drawing Conclusions.**

45. B. The information comes from a government agency called the FDA, and government sources are credible. **Skill: Understanding Primary Sources, Making Inferences, and Drawing Conclusions.**

46. B. One way to verify facts is to call all the numbers of the government agencies listed at the bottom of the page for more information. **Skill: Understanding Primary Sources, Making Inferences, and Drawing Conclusions.**

47. D. Highly edited videos can be biased because parts could be purposely removed. **Skill: Understanding Primary Sources, Making Inferences, and Drawing Conclusions.**

Section III. Vocabulary & General Knowledge

1. B. The root word *spher* means "ball-like," so spherical means round. **Skill: Root Words, Prefixes, and Suffixes.**

2. D. The root *veter* means "old," as in the word *veteran*. **Skill: Root Words, Prefixes, and Suffixes.**

3. D. The root word *therm* means "heat, or warm," so endotherm is a warm-blooded animal. **Skill: Root Words, Prefixes, and Suffixes.**

4. A. The suffix that means "more" is *-er* as in the word *warmer*. **Skill: Root Words, Prefixes, and Suffixes.**

5. B. The root that means "truth" is *ver* as in the word *verify*. **Skill: Root Words, Prefixes, and Suffixes.**

6. D. The prefix that means "false" is *pseudo-* as in the word *pseudonym*. **Skill: Root Words, Prefixes, and Suffixes.**

7. C. The prefix *tri* -means "three," so a tripod would be a stand with three legs. **Skill: Root Words, Prefixes, and Suffixes.**

8. B. The root word *fal* means "false," and the suffix *-ible* means "able to," so fallible means "capable of making errors." **Skill: Root Words, Prefixes, and Suffixes.**

9. A. The root word *terr* means "earth," and the prefix *extra-* means "beyond," so extraterrestrial beings are ones that are not of this earth. **Skill: Root Words, Prefixes, and Suffixes.**

10. D. The root *syn* means "same," and *chron* means "time," so to synchronize means "to cause to occur at the same time." **Skill: Root Words, Prefixes, and Suffixes.**

11. A. The suffix that means "younger or inferior" is *-ling* as in *duckling*. **Skill: Root Words, Prefixes, and Suffixes.**

12. D. The root that means "self" is *auto* as in the word *autobiography*. **Skill: Root Words, Prefixes, and Suffixes.**

13. B. The prefix that means "between" is *intra-* as in the word *intramural*. **Skill: Root Words, Prefixes, and Suffixes.**

14. D. The word "track" has more than one meaning. **Skill: Context Clues and Multiple Meaning Words.**

15. B. The meaning of <u>crack</u> in the context of this sentence is "a sudden sharp and loud noise." **Skill: Context Clues and Multiple Meaning Words.**

16. B. The meaning of <u>court</u> in this context is "a royal household or entourage." The phrase "group" helps you figure out which meaning of <u>court</u> is being used. **Skill: Context Clues and Multiple Meaning Words.**

17. A. The meaning of <u>omnipotent</u> in the context of this sentence is "almighty." **Skill: Context Clues and Multiple Meaning Words.**

18. C. The meaning of <u>ornate</u> in this context is "highly decorated." The phrase "detail" helps you figure out the meaning of <u>ornate</u>. **Skill: Context Clues and Multiple Meaning Words.**

19. D. The word "nursery" has more than one meaning. **Skill: Context Clues and Multiple Meaning Words.**

20. A. The meaning of <u>review</u> in the context of this sentence is "critique." **Skill: Context Clues and Multiple Meaning Words.**

21. B. The meaning of <u>spring</u> in this context is "to move or jump quickly upward and forward." The phrase "out of" helps you figure out which meaning of <u>spring</u> is being used. **Skill: Context Clues and Multiple Meaning Words.**

22. C. The meaning of <u>petulant</u> in the context of this sentence is "irritable." **Skill: Context Clues and Multiple Meaning Words.**

23. B. The meaning of <u>prohibit</u> in this context is "outlaw." The word "forbidden" helps you figure out the meaning of <u>prohibit</u>. **Skill: Context Clues and Multiple Meaning Words.**

24. B. The word "minor" has more than one meaning. **Skill: Context Clues and Multiple Meaning Words.**

25. D. The meaning of <u>signal</u> in the context of this sentence is "an electrical impulse." **Skill: Context Clues and Multiple Meaning Words.**

26. A. The meaning of <u>jerk</u> in this context is "obnoxious." The phrase "contempt" helps you figure out which meaning of <u>jerk</u> is being used. **Skill: Context Clues and Multiple Meaning Words.**

27. A. The meaning of <u>scorn</u> in the context of this sentence is "deride." **Skill: Context Clues and Multiple Meaning Words.**

28. B. The meaning of <u>ubiquitous</u> in this context is "being everywhere at once." The phrase "commonly seen" helps you figure out the meaning of <u>ubiquitous</u>. **Skill: Context Clues and Multiple Meaning Words.**

29. A. The word "master" has more than one meaning. **Skill: Context Clues and Multiple Meaning Words.**

30. C. The meaning of <u>break</u> in the context of this sentence is "get change." **Skill: Context Clues and Multiple Meaning Words.**

31. B. The meaning of <u>flourish</u> in the context of this sentence is "grow." **Skill: Context Clues and Multiple Meaning Words.**

32. B. The meaning of <u>scale</u> in this context is "to climb." The word "fence" help you figure out which meaning of <u>scale</u> is being used. **Skill: Context Clues and Multiple Meaning Words.**

33. A. The meaning of <u>interest</u> in the context of this sentence is "profit." **Skill: Context Clues and Multiple Meaning Words.**

34. A. The meaning of <u>competent</u> in the context of this sentence is "skilled." **Skill: Context Clues and Multiple Meaning Words.**

35. C. The root word that means "hearing" is "audi." **Skill: Domain-Specific Words: Medical Industry.**

36. A. "Osteo" refers to the "bones" so the surgeon was going to operate on the patient's bone. **Skill: Domain-Specific Words: Medical Industry.**

37. B. "Oncology" is the study and treatment of tumors. **Skill: Domain-Specific Words: Medical Industry.**

38. A. The suffix –asthenia means "weakness." **Skill: Domain-Specific Words: Medical Industry.**

39. B. The word "hysterectomy" means "removal of the uterus" because "hyster" pertains to a womb and "ectomy" means "removal of." **Skill: Domain-Specific Words: Medical Industry.**

40. D. Adding the suffix "metry" meaning "measuring" would make the word "pelvimetry," or taking measurements of the pelvis. **Skill: Domain-Specific Words: Medical Industry.**

41. B. A "pulmonary" issue would be one involving the lungs. **Skill: Domain-Specific Words: Medical Industry.**

42. C. "Rhin" pertains to the nose, so the patient's nose was hurting. **Skill: Domain-Specific Words: Medical Industry.**

43. D. The suffix "stomy" would make the word "tracheostomy" to complete the sentence. **Skill: Domain-Specific Words: Medical Industry.**

44. D. "Hydrotherapy" means "treatment with water." **Skill: Domain-Specific Words: Medical Industry.**

45. B. The root word that means "sugar" is "glyc." **Skill: Domain-Specific Words: Medical Industry.**

46. D. "Encephal" refers to the "brain," so the patient was suffering from inflammation of the brain. **Skill: Domain-Specific Words: Medical Industry.**

47. B. "Hepatology" is the study of the liver, gallbladder, and pancreas. **Skill: Domain-Specific Words: Medical Industry.**

48. A. The suffix –genic means "causing" as in the word "carcinogenic," which means "cancer causing." **Skill: Domain-Specific Words: Medical Industry.**

49. D. The word "neuroplasty" means the surgical repair of a nerve because "neuro" means "nerve" and "plasty" means "surgical repair of." **Skill: Domain-Specific Words: Medical Industry.**

50. C. Adding the prefix "peri" meaning "surrounding" would make the word "perinatal," or the word describing the time and events surrounding both before and after a birth. **Skill: Domain-Specific Words: Medical Industry.**

Section IV. Grammar

1. B. *Business* is the only correct spelling. **Skill: Spelling.**

2. A. *Argument* is the only correct spelling. **Skill: Spelling.**

3. B. *Criticism* is the only correct spelling. **Skill: Spelling.**

4. D. *Commitment* is the only one spelled correctly. **Skill: Spelling.**

5. D. *december, she, and christmas.* All months and holidays are capitalized. *She* is the beginning of a sentence and needs to be capitalized. **Skill: Capitalization.**

6. D. *she, do, and indian. She* is at the beginning of the sentence and needs to be capitalized. *Do* is at the beginning of a quoted sentence and also needs to be capitalized. Nationalities such as Indian should always be capitalized. **Skill: Capitalization.**

7. D. *new york, los angeles, and chicago.* All names of cities should be capitalized. **Skill: Capitalization.**

8. A. *on and wednesdays.* The first word of the sentence and all days of the week need to be capitalized. *Month* and *exterminator* are general terms and do not need to be capitalized. **Skill: Capitalization.**

9. C. *No, I am not leaving yet.* Commas are used after yes or no. **Skill: Punctuation.**

10. C. *JFK said, "Ask not what your country can do for you; ask what you can do for your country."* Quotation marks enclose words or sentences that someone else said or wrote. **Skill: Punctuation.**

11. A. *Wait!* Exclamation points are placed at the end of a sentence and indicate strong feelings, shouting, or emphasis. **Skill: Punctuation.**

12. A. *It was good, wasn't it?* Commas are used before question tags. **Skill: Punctuation.**

13. D. *Health* is an abstract noun; it does not physically exist. **Skill: Nouns.**

14. D. The noun is *uncle.* **Skill: Nouns.**

15. D. *Pearl S. Buck* is the subject of this sentence. **Skill: Nouns.**

16. C. *Children* is a plural noun. **Skill: Nouns.**

17. D. *Yours* is a possessive pronoun. **Skill: Pronouns.**

18. D. We are looking for a possessive pronoun. *Whose* is a relative pronoun and can only be used to show possession when the sentence is a question. **Skill: Pronouns.**

19. B. A subject pronoun must be used. **Skill: Pronouns.**

20. C. *Red* is an adjective that describes the noun *roses.* **Skill: Adjectives and Adverbs.**

21. D. *So* is an adverb that describes the adjective *upsetting.* **Skill: Adjectives and Adverbs.**

22. D. *Talented* is an adjective that describes the noun *gymnast.* **Skill: Adjectives and Adverbs.**

23. C. *Late* is an adjective that describes the noun *flight.* **Skill: Adjectives and Adverbs.**

24. C. *And* is a conjunction. **Skill: Conjunctions and Prepositions.**

25. A. *It* is a pronoun, not a preposition. **Skill: Conjunctions and Prepositions.**

26. A. *Yikes* is an interjection. **Skill: Conjunctions and Prepositions.**

27. C. *At* is a preposition. **Skill: Conjunctions and Prepositions.**

28. B. *Were grabbing* is past progressive, and *broke* is simple past. **Skill: Verbs and Verb Tenses.**

29. C. *Rises* is a verb. **Skill: Verbs and Verb Tenses.**

30. A. *Ran* is the main verb, and there is not a helping verb in this sentence. **Skill: Verbs and Verb Tenses.**

31. C. *The automobile* and *the personal computer* are both singular subjects connected by *or*, so they take a singular verb form. **Skill: Subject and Verb Agreement.**

32. B. The verb *wants* has the subject *she.* **Skill: Subject and Verb Agreement.**

33. B. The word *its* is the possessive for *it.* It is not a verb. **Skill: Subject and Verb Agreement.**

34. C. The verb *honor* must agree with the subject *Americans.* **Skill: Subject and Verb Agreement.**

35. C. This option would make the sentence a compound sentence. **Skill: Types of Sentences.**

36. D. The subordinate conjunction "because" combines the sentences and puts the focus on Tony preparing for his job interview. **Skill: Types of Sentences.**

37. D. This sentence correctly fixes the run-on sentence. **Skill: Types of Sentences.**

38. A. The subordinate conjunction "since" combines the sentences and puts the focus on the people relocating to save money. **Skill: Types of Sentences.**

39. B. The couple went on a stroll through the park. It is independent because it has a subject, verb, and expresses a complete thought. **Skill: Types of Clauses.**

40. C. People do not exercise as much as they should. It is independent because it has a subject, verb, and expresses a complete thought. **Skill: Types of Clauses.**

41. A. When I lived in New York City. It is dependent because it does not express a complete thought and relies on the independent clause. The word "when" also signifies the beginning of a dependent clause. **Skill: Types of Clauses.**

42. A. While her kids swam in the pool. It is dependent because it does not express a complete thought and relies on the independent clause. The word "while" also signifies the beginning of a dependent clause. **Skill: Types of Clauses.**

43. D. *Closely* is a modifier; it is an adverb that describes *following.* **Skill: Modifiers.**

44. B. *Woman* is not a modifier. **Skill: Modifiers.**

45. A. *Black* is a modifier; it is an adjective that describes *dog.* **Skill: Modifiers.**

46. B. The adjective *great* describes *time.* **Skill: Modifiers.**

47. D. *Candles* is the direct object of the verb *held.* **Skill: Direct Objects and Indirect Objects.**

48. C. *The dog* is the direct object of the verb *walk.* **Skill: Direct Objects and Indirect Objects.**

49. D. *The road* is a direct object of the verb *cross.* **Skill: Direct Objects and Indirect Objects.**

50. C. *The moon* is the object of the preposition *on.* **Skill: Direct Objects and Indirect Objects.**

Section V. Biology

1. B. The researcher is collecting qualitative data by describing what happens to the plant under specific conditions. This data collection corresponds to the observation step of the scientific method. **Skill: An Introduction to Biology.**

2. C. Adenine and thymine bond with each other to form a nucleotide. This nucleotide is the monomer of the nucleic acid DNA. **Skill: An Introduction to Biology.**

3. B. Lipid synthesis is anabolic because monomers like fatty acids are used to synthesize lipid molecules. **Skill: An Introduction to Biology.**

4. C. Metabolic reactions are cyclic, which means they keep occurring as long as enough starting materials are available to allow the reaction to proceed. **Skill: An Introduction to Biology.**

5. A. Whenever a new living thing is discovered or identified, it needs to be classified and named. A taxonomic system can be used to do this. **Skill: An Introduction to Biology.**

6. C. Hydrogen bonding is a type of weak attraction that forms between water molecules. **Skill: An Introduction to Biology.**

7. D. Each level is found in the level above it. The levels above class are phylum and kingdom. **Skill: An Introduction to Biology.**

8. D. Because a cell membrane is selectively permeable, only certain molecules are allowed to enter. For molecules such as sodium ions to enter, they have to travel through specialized channels. **Skill: Cell Structure, Function, and Type.**

9. C. The cell wall provides structural support and protects the cell from the external environment. The cell membrane is selectively permeable, allowing only certain things from the outside environment to enter. **Skill: Cell Structure, Function, and Type.**

10. B. Heterotrophs such as bears are organisms that function as consumers and ingest food as an energy source. **Skill: Cell Structure, Function, and Type.**

11. C. A consumer is any living thing that must consume or feed on another living thing to obtain energy. A consumer is also known as a heterotroph. **Skill: Cell Structure, Function, and Type.**

12. B. The chloroplast traps sunlight energy for a plant cell to make food via photosynthesis. Mitochondria convert stored energy from food into a usable form that the cell can use. **Skill: Cell Structure, Function, and Type.**

13. A. After scientists were able to view cells under the microscope they formulated the cell theory. One part of this theory concluded that all cells are alive. They also represent the basic unit of life. **Skill: Cell Structure Function and Type**

14. D. The ATP provides the reducing power to make carbon dioxide into sugar. **Skill: Cellular Reproduction, Cellular Respiration, and Photosynthesis.**

15. D. Plants use cell plates to divide a cell after the cell has completed mitosis. This physical separation of one cell into two is known as cytokinesis. **Skill: Cellular Reproduction, Cellular Respiration, and Photosynthesis.**

16. A. A cell produces energy through metabolism by breaking glucose molecules into pyruvate. This happens via glycolysis. The pyruvate molecule is prepped for the citric acid cycle by being oxidized to acetyl-CoA. Once the citric acid cycle happens, the largest amount of energy is generated via the electron transport chain. **Skill: Cellular Reproduction, Cellular Respiration, and Photosynthesis.**

17. A. Before mitosis or meiosis occurs, interphase must happen. This is when the cell cycle takes place. **Skill: Cellular Reproduction, Cellular Respiration, and Photosynthesis.**

18. B. The final process in cellular respiration, the electron transport chain, yields the largest amount of ATP for a cell. Chemiosmosis, which involves the creation of a proton gradient (with the help of NADH and FADH), is part of this step for cellular respiration. **Skill: Cellular Reproduction, Cellular Respiration, and Photosynthesis.**

19. D. Cell reproduction is the process where cells grow and differentiate to create offspring or new cells. When the skin is damaged, new skin cells are needed which are created through cell reproduction. **Skill: Cellular Reproduction, Cellular Respiration, and Photosynthesis**

20. C. Peptide bonds connect amino acids together to form a protein. **Skill: Genetics and DNA.**

21. A. Translation produces short sequences of proteins called amino acids. **Skill: Genetics and DNA.**

22. C. The RNA polymerase functions as an enzyme. **Skill: Genetics and DNA.**

23. A. A DNA molecule and its associated proteins coil tightly right before cellular division. **Skill: Genetics and DNA.**

24. A. The protein disc that connects the two chromatids is the centromere. **Skill: Genetics and DNA.**

25. B. Mendel was accurately able to predict the patterns of heredity by studying rules related to genetics. These rules helped shape his theory of heredity. **Skill: Genetics and DNA.**

Section VI. Chemistry

1. A. The mass of an object is determined by using a balance. Electric balances are used to measure a very small mass. **Skill: Designing an Experiment.**

2. B. The independent variable is the administered drug because it is being manipulated in the experiment. The condition, following treatment with the drug, is the dependent variable. Condition is a type of response that is dependent on the drug being administered. **Skill: Designing an Experiment.**

3. B. The plant left outside is the control because it is not influenced by the independent variable, which is not experimentally manipulated. **Skill: Designing an Experiment.**

4. C. Deductive reasoning uses a "from the top down" approach and includes making predictions from a general idea to create a conclusion. **Skill: Designing an Experiment.**

5. B. Both atoms can be identified as neon because the atomic number, which equals the number of protons, is 10 for both. However, they have different masses. The mass of Atom Y can be determined by adding the numbers of protons and neutrons (10 + 12) to get 22, which is

different from the mass of Atom X. Because they are the same element with different masses, Atom X and Atom Y are isotopes. **Skill: Scientific Notation.**

6. A. The atomic number for tin is 50, which means all atoms of tin have 50 protons. To determine the number of neutrons, subtract the number of protons from the mass number: 120 – 50 = 70 neutrons. Because the atom is neutral, it has 50 electrons to balance the charge of the protons. **Skill: Scientific Notation.**

7. A. In a neutral atom, the number of electrons is equal to the number of protons. Because the atomic number of iodine is 53, there are 53 protons and 53 electrons to balance the charge. **Skill: Scientific Notation.**

8. B. The number of protons, 28, gives the atomic number, which identifies this atom as nickel. The mass is the number after the dash in the isotope name, which is determined by adding the numbers of protons and neutrons (28 + 32 = 60). **Skill: Scientific Notation.**

9. B. There are 1,000 grams in 1 kilogram. This means 1,800 grams divided by 1,000 grams yields 1.8 kilograms. **Skill: Temperature and the Metric System.**

10. D. There are 2 cups in 1 pint. Thus, 22 pints is 44 cups. **Skill: Temperature and the Metric System.**

11. B. There are 2.54 centimeters in 1 inch. Dividing 35 by 2.54 converts 35 centimeters to 13.77 inches. **Skill: Temperature and the Metric System.**

12. B. There are $\frac{1}{100}$, or 0.01 grams, in 1 centigram. A gram is larger than a centigram. **Skill: Temperature and the Metric System.**

13. A. During deposition, a gas turns to a solid. The particles will have less energy as a solid at the end of the phase change than as a gas at the beginning. **Skill: States of Matter.**

14. B. Any substance will condense and boil at the same temperature, assuming these processes are carried out under the same conditions. This is the temperature at which the substance transitions between liquid and gas states. **Skill: States of Matter.**

15. B. As particles condense, the substance turns from gas to liquid. The particles of liquids are closer together than the particles of gas. **Skill: States of Matter.**

16. B. Evaporation occurs on the surface of a substance, and boiling occurs throughout a substance. **Skill: Properties of Matter.**

17. C. Freezing is the change of a liquid to a solid. **Skill: Properties of Matter.**

18. C. Electrons in the third shell are the valence electrons for this atom, which are the electrons involved in bonding. **Skill: Chemical Bonds.**

19. B. To become stable, a potassium atom will lose one electron to form an ion with a +1 charge, and a nitrogen atom will gain three electrons to form an ion with a -3 charge. Because ionic compounds are neutral, it will require three potassium ions to balance the charge of one nitrogen ion. **Skill: Chemical Bonds.**

20. B. The net charge is zero for any ionic compound because the positive charge of the cation balances the negative charge of the anion. For barium iodide, the barium cation has a charge of +2 and is balanced by two iodide ions. Because each iodide ion has a charge of -1, the total negative charge provided by the two iodide ions is -2. **Skill: Chemical Bonds.**

21. C. Sodium replaces zinc in the compound zinc chloride ($ZnCl_2$), which produces a new compound, sodium chloride (NaCl), and zinc metal. **Skill: Chemical Solutions.**

22. D. In this reaction, two aqueous solutions are mixed, which means that all species are dissolved in water. This forms a solution, which is a type of heterogeneous mixture. After the reaction occurs, a solid product is formed, while the other product remains in solution, dissolved in water. Because the solid product is visibly separate from the solution, this is a heterogeneous mixture. **Skill: Chemical Solutions.**

23. B. The conjugate base is NO_2^- because the acid HNO_2 donates a hydrogen ion during the reaction. **Skill: Acids and Bases.**

24. D. Nitric acid (HNO_3) reacts with sodium hydroxide (NaOH) in a neutralization reaction to form $NaNO_3$ and water (H_2O). **Skill: Acids and Bases.**

25. B. Hydrochloric acid, HCl, is a strong acid because it is able to fully ionize, contributing its maximum number of ions in solution. **Skill: Acids and Bases.**

Section VII. Anatomy & Physiology

1. B. The midsagittal plane divides the body into two equal parts. **Skill: Organization of the Human Body.**

2. B. Homeostasis is the steady, optimal condition of a human body. **Skill: Organization of the Human Body.**

3. D. Blood is responsible for transporting waste products to the liver, where they are excreted as bile from the liver or as urine by the kidneys. **Skill: Cardiovascular System.**

4. A. Blood flows in one direction when it leaves the aorta and travels through the arteries. **Skill: Cardiovascular System.**

5. D. Epithelial mucosal cells that line the nose secrete mucous as a defense mechanism to prevent particles from entering the lungs. **Skill: The Respiratory System.**

6. D. Alveoli are tiny air sacs found within the lungs. They have large surface areas and are the sites for gas exchange. **Skill: The Respiratory System.**

7. D. The cardiac sphincter opens for food to enter the stomach. **Skill: Gastrointestinal System.**

8. A. Glycerol is one of the end products of lipid breakdown. Therefore, it is small enough to diffuse through the lining of the small intestine. **Skill: Gastrointestinal System.**

9. A. The uterus, cervix, Fallopian tube, ovaries, and vagina are components of the female reproductive system; the epididymis, corpus cavernosum, and prostate gland are components of the male reproductive system. **Skill: Reproductive System.**

10. C. Humans utilize sexual reproduction. **Skill: Reproductive System.**

11. C. The renal tubule consists of the proximal and distal convoluted tubules, loop of Henle, and collecting duct. The renal tubule terminates at the tip of the medullary pyramid. Its attachment begins at the glomerulus. **Skill: The Urinary System.**

12. B. With help from the kidneys and the hormone ADH, the urinary system regulates the quantity of water that is lost due to blood filtration. **Skill: The Urinary System.**

13. A. Ossification is the process of generating new bone tissue by filling in cartilage with mineral deposits to harden the cartilage. Growth plates are present near the ends of long bones. They are sites where ossification occurs so that a child's long bones can grow and the child can get taller. **Skill: Skeletal System.**

14. A. Bone resorption is a process that dissolves old bone tissue so that it can undergo remodeling to produce new bone tissue. When bones dissolve during the resorption process, minerals stored in reservoirs of bone are released and pushed through circulation for use. **Skill: Skeletal System.**

15. B. Skeletal muscle cells have an elongated shape. These muscle cells are striated and under voluntary control. **Skill: Muscular System.**

16. C. Ligaments are structures that attach bone to bone. They allow less movement than other structures like joints. **Skill: Muscular System.**

17. A. When a flexor muscle contracts, it causes a joint to bend. During this contraction, the extension muscle straightens, or elongates. **Skill: Muscular System.**

18. A. The dermis is the second layer of the skin, located under the epidermis. This layer contains blood vessels and nerve endings, which enable a person to feel sensations on the skin. **Skill: Integumentary System.**

19. C. The skin has three layers: epidermis, dermis, and subcutaneous tissue layer. The epidermis is made of four or five layers. **Skill: Integumentary System.**

20. C. The limbic system is part of the forebrain, or cerebrum. It consists of four major structures: hypothalamus, hippocampus, amygdala, and thalamus. **Skill: The Nervous System.**

21. C. Smell is the only sense that bypasses the thalamus during external signal processing by the CNS. The thalamus is the structure of the limbic system that directly receives sensory information from nerves. **Skill: The Nervous System.**

22. B. Because muscle density decreases as a result of hormonal changes due to aging, strength would decrease. **Skill: Endocrine System.**

23. B. A decreased metabolic rate would promote weight gain. **Skill: Endocrine System.**

24. D. The HIV virus can recognize a human cell surface receptor on certain immune system cells, primarily the macrophages and helper T cells. This enables it to destroy these cells. **Skill: The Lymphatic System.**

25. D. Rheumatoid arthritis is an autoimmune disease. **Skill: The Lymphatic System.**

Section VIII. Physics

1. B. Consistently measuring time requires a process that is consistently periodic. Only the phases of the moon occur at regular intervals. **Skill: Nature of Motion.**

2. B. Use Newton's second law of motion: $F = ma$. (Vectors are unnecessary because the problem only deals with scalars.) Plug in the numbers and solve for a, noting that it will be in meters per square second.

$$F = ma$$

$$144 \text{ N} = (2.0 \text{ kg})a$$

$$a = \frac{144 \text{ N}}{2.0 \text{ kg}} = 72 \text{ m/s}^2$$

Skill: Nature of Motion.

3. B. Using Newton's second law of motion, the net force on an object produces an acceleration commensurate with its mass: $\vec{F} = m\vec{a}$. Note that because the force and acceleration must be in the same direction to maintain this equality, the acceleration must be southward. Dealing only in magnitudes, $F = ma$. Thus,

$$a = \frac{F}{m} = \frac{75 \text{ N}}{3.0 \text{ kg}} = 25 \text{ m/s}^2$$

Skill: Nature of Motion.

4. D. One way to check is to pick two different vectors (e.g., $\vec{a} = (2, 3)$ and $\vec{b} = (1, 4)$) and a scalar (e.g., $c = 5$) and plug them into each expression. The equalities will not hold in answers A, B, and C. Alternatively, note that because vector addition is commutative, $\vec{a} + \vec{b} = \vec{b} + \vec{a}$ is always true. **Skill: Nature of Motion.**

5. D. The speed of a moving object is the magnitude (or length) of its velocity—in this case, the magnitude of (−2.12, 6.37) in meters per second.

$$\sqrt{(-2.12)^2 + (6.37)^2} = \sqrt{4.49 + 40.6} = \sqrt{45.1} = 6.72$$

Skill: Nature of Motion.

6. D. Draw a circle and indicate the direction of motion as counterclockwise. The centripetal acceleration always directed toward the center; it points south at the top (northernmost) point of the circle. At that point, if the child jumps off, he experiences no more acceleration and maintains the horizontal velocity he had when he jumped. That velocity is directed west. **Skill: Friction.**

7. D. If the passenger feels a force pushing forward or backward, the car is just decelerating or accelerating along a line, regardless of whether that force is constant or changing in magnitude. That type of motion is linear. If the passenger feels a force to either side, the car is turning in one direction or the other, meaning its motion is nonlinear. Whether the force is increasing or decreasing is unimportant to this experiment. **Skill: Friction.**

8. B. If the driver does nothing, his car will lose speed, eventually coming to a stop. Because the friction force is opposite in direction to the velocity, hitting the gas pedal will apply an additional force in the direction of the velocity to cancel the friction. **Skill: Friction.**

9. A. The centrifugal force is a ghost force, but it is equal in magnitude (but opposite in direction) to the centripetal force. Because a force is the mass times the acceleration, the plane's centripetal acceleration (which is also the passenger's centripetal acceleration) is the magnitude of the centrifugal force divided by the mass of the passenger.

$$F_c = m a_c$$
$$a_c = \frac{F_c}{m} = \frac{25\,\text{N}}{65\,\text{kg}} = 0.38 \text{ m/s}^2$$

Skill: Friction.

10. D. The angular frequency (ω), the frequency (f), and the period (T) are all directly related:

$$\omega = 2\pi f = \frac{2\pi}{T}$$

The centripetal acceleration, however, is also dependent on the radius of the circle, so it can vary independently of the other three parameters. **Skill: Friction.**

11. B. The speed of mechanical waves depends on the medium's (material's) compressibility and density. If the compressibility is the same in materials X and Y, then the speed depends solely on the density. Because waves travel faster in denser materials, statement B is correct. **Skill: Waves and Sounds.**

12. A. The nucleus of an atom is made of protons and neutrons. Electrons "orbit" the nucleus. **Skill: Waves and Sounds.**

13. A. Optics is the study of light, often using a ray representation. Only choice A involves light (electromagnetic waves). The others involve mechanical waves. **Skill: Waves and Sounds.**

14. A. A ray that hits a mirror at 0° to the normal is following the normal line. If the two mirrors are parallel and facing each other, the normal of one mirror is the same as the normal for the other. The ray will therefore bounce back and forth along the normal line between the two mirrors, meaning the angle of reflection will always be 0° from the normal. **Skill: Waves and Sounds.**

15. D. The wave speed v is related to the frequency f and wavelength λ by the formula $v = \lambda f$. Multiply the frequency (which is in hertz, or inverse seconds) by the wavelength to get the wave speed in feet per second. **Skill: Waves and Sounds.**

16. A. Use the universal gravitation formula to solve. Then, plug in all known variables and calculate.

$$F = G\left(\frac{m_1 \cdot m_2}{r^2}\right)$$

$$F = \left(6.67 \times 10^{-11}\,\frac{N \cdot m^2}{kg^2}\right)\left(\frac{2{,}031{,}000\text{ kg} \cdot 11{,}110\text{ kg}}{(50.0\text{ m})^2}\right)$$

$$F = 6.02 \times 10^{-4}\,N$$

Skill: Kinetic Energy.

17. C. Use the formula for momentum to solve for m. Then, plug in all known variables and calculate.

$$\rho = mv$$

$$m = \frac{\rho}{v}$$

$$m = \frac{300{,}000\,\frac{kg \cdot m}{s}}{15\frac{m}{s}}$$

$$m = 20{,}000\text{ kg}$$

Skill: Kinetic Energy.

18. B. Use the impulse-momentum theorem and solve for mass. Then, plug in all known variables and calculate. Convert the answer from kilograms to grams. **Skill: Kinetic Energy.**

$$F\Delta t = mv$$

$$m = \frac{F\Delta t}{v}$$

$$m = \frac{(12\ N)(0.20\ s)}{101\ \frac{m}{s}}$$

$$m = 0.024\ \text{kg}$$

$$m = 24\ \text{g}$$

Skill: Kinetic Energy.

19. D. Use the potential energy formula to solve for h. Convert mass from grams to kilograms. Then, plug in all known variables and calculate.

$$PE = mgh$$

$$h = \frac{PE}{mg}$$

$$h = \frac{0.27\ J}{(0.055\ \text{kg})\left(9.8\ \frac{m}{s^2}\right)}$$

$$h = 0.50\ m$$

Skill: Kinetic Energy.

20. D. Use the formula for momentum to solve. Convert the mass to kilograms. Then, plug in all known variables and calculate.

$$\rho = mv$$

$$\rho = (0.0459\ \text{kg})\left(81\ \frac{m}{s}\right)$$

$$\rho = 3.7\ \frac{\text{kg} \cdot \text{m}}{\text{s}}$$

Skill: Kinetic Energy.

21. B. An electric current is moving charge. Because electrons have an electric charge, they create an electric current when they move. **Skill: Electricity and Magnetism.**

22. C. Consider any point in the circuit between the battery's positive and negative terminals: the current going into that point must equal the current coming out of it. In this case, that means the current everywhere—including at the negative battery terminal—must be the same, 0.001 amps. **Skill: Electricity and Magnetism.**

23. A. Halfway between any two equally charged objects, the force from one object is equal in magnitude but opposite in direction to the force from the other object. These forces cancel, so the field is 0. **Skill: Electricity and Magnetism.**

24. D. Using Ohm's law:

$V = IR$

$R = \frac{V}{I} = \frac{5.0 \text{ volts}}{0.020 \text{ amps}} = 250 \text{ ohms}$

Skill: Electricity and Magnetism.

25. B. Use Ohm's law:

$V = IR$

$V = (0.01 \text{ amps}) \times (100 \text{ ohms}) = 1 \text{ volt}$

Skill: Electricity and Magnetism.

HESI Practice Exam 2

Section I. Mathematics

You have 50 minutes to complete 50 questions.

1. Which procedure is impossible?

   A. Adding two negative numbers

   B. Subtracting a negative number from zero

   C. Adding two quantities with different units

   D. Placing negative numbers on the number line

2. What is 0 − 561?

   A. 561   C. −561

   B. 0   D. −1,122

3. Which mathematical statement is true?

   A. 6 > 9   C. 18 < −35

   B. −3 > 2   D. 20 > −21

4. What is 743 − 744?

   A. −1   C. 1

   B. 0   D. 1,487

5. How many numbers are on the complete number line?

   A. 7   C. 1,000,000

   B. 100   D. None of the above

6. Evaluate the expression

   (3 × (4 + 9) ÷ 13 − 2) + 1.

   A. −2   C. 2

   B. 0   D. 5

7. Evaluate the expression 8 × 15.

   A. 85   C. 115

   B. 105   D. 120

8. Evaluate the expression (−20) ÷ (−5).

   A. −5   C. 4

   B. −4   D. 5

9. Given an expression with no parentheses, which should be evaluated first?

   A. Division   C. Subtraction

   B. Addition   D. Any of the above

10. If a certain widget sells for $5 each and Linda has $321, how many widgets can she buy?

    A. 1   C. 65

    B. 64   D. 1,605

11. Which decimal is the greatest?

    A. 1.7805   C. 1.7085

    B. 1.5807   D. 1.8057

12. Change 0.375 to a fraction. Simplify completely.

    A. $\frac{3}{8}$ C. $\frac{1}{2}$

    B. $\frac{2}{5}$ D. $\frac{7}{16}$

13. Change 2.5 to a fraction. Simplify completely.

    A. $2\frac{1}{8}$ C. $2\frac{1}{3}$

    B. $2\frac{1}{4}$ D. $2\frac{1}{2}$

14. Write 12.5% as a fraction.

    A. $\frac{1}{12}$ C. $\frac{1}{8}$

    B. $\frac{1}{9}$ D. $\frac{1}{7}$

15. Write 145.5% as a decimal.

    A. 1.455   C. 145.5

    B. 14.55   D. 1455

16. Solve the equation for the unknown,
    $a-10 = -20$.

    A. -30 C. 2

    B. -10 D. 200

17. Solve the equation for the unknown x,
    $y = mx + b$.

    A. $y-bm = x$ C. $\frac{y-b}{m} = x$

    B. $y + bm = x$ D. $\frac{y+b}{m} = x$

18. Solve the inequality for the unknown,
    $\frac{1}{2}(4x + 3) < \frac{3}{4}x + 2$.

    A. $x < \frac{2}{5}$ C. $x < \frac{6}{5}$

    B. $x > \frac{2}{5}$ D. $x > \frac{6}{5}$

19. Solve the equation for the unknown,
    $\frac{1}{3}(3x + 2) + 3 = 2x + 3$.

    A. -4 C. $\frac{2}{3}$

    B. $-\frac{2}{3}$ D. 4

20. Solve the system of equations, $\begin{array}{l} y = -2x \\ x^2 + y^2 = 5 \end{array}$.

    A. (1, -2) and (-1, 2)

    B. (1, 2) and (-1, -2)

    C. (2, -1) and (-2, 1)

    D. (2, 1) and (-2, -1)

21. Solve the system of equations,
    $\begin{array}{l} y = 4x \\ x^2 + y^2 = 17 \end{array}$.

    A. (4, 1) and (-4, -1)

    B. (-4, 1) and (4, -1)

    C. (-1, 4) and (1, -4)

    D. (1, 4) and (-1, -4)

22. Solve the system of equations,
    $\begin{array}{l} y = -3x \\ x^2 + y^2 = 20 \end{array}$.

    A. (1.4, 4.2) and (-1.4, -4.2)

    B. (-1.4, 4.2) and (1.4, -4.2)

    C. (-2, 6) and (2, -6)

    D. (2, 6) and (-2, -6)

23. Solve the system of equations,
    $\begin{array}{l} 5x + 3y = 22 \\ 2x-5y = -16 \end{array}$.

    A. (2, 4)   C. (-2, -3)

    B. (4, 2)   D. (-3, -2)

24. Divide $1\frac{2}{3} \div 3\frac{7}{12}$.

    A. $\frac{20}{43}$ C. $3\frac{3}{4}$

    B. $3\frac{7}{18}$ D. $5\frac{35}{36}$

25. Multiply $2\frac{1}{2} \times 3\frac{3}{4}$.

    A. $5\frac{3}{8}$ C. $7\frac{3}{8}$

    B. $6\frac{3}{8}$ D. $9\frac{3}{8}$

26. Divide $1\frac{6}{7} \div \frac{3}{14}$.

    A. $\frac{39}{91}$ C. $7\frac{1}{14}$

    B. $1\frac{1}{2}$ D. $8\frac{2}{3}$

27. Multiply $3\frac{1}{4} \times 2\frac{2}{3}$.

    A. $6\frac{1}{2}$ C. $8\frac{1}{2}$

    B. $6\frac{2}{3}$ D. $8\frac{2}{3}$

28. Perform the operation,
$(3y^3-4y^2 + 6y + 3)-(2y^3-3y)$.

   A. $5y^3-4y^2 + 3y + 3$

   B. $y^3-4y^2 + 3y + 3$

   C. $5y^3-4y^2 + 9y + 3$

   D. $y^3-4y^2 + 9y + 3$

29. Multiply, $(2xy-1)(3xy-2)$.

   A. $6x^2y^2 + xy + 2$

   B. $6x^2y^2-xy + 2$

   C. $6x^2y^2 + 7xy + 2$

   D. $6x^2y^2-7xy + 2$

30. Perform the operation,
$(8x + 2xy-4y) + (-7x-3xy + 2y)$.

   A. $x + xy-2y$

   B. $x-xy-2y$

   C. $x-xy + 2y$

   D. $x + xy + 2y$

31. Perform the operation,
$(3y^2 + 4y)-(5y^3-2y^2 + 3)$.

   A. $-5y^3 + y^2 + 4y-3$

   B. $-5y^3 + 5y^2 + 4y + 3$

   C. $-5y^3 + y^2 + 4y + 3$

   D. $-5y^3 + 5y^2 + 4y-3$

32. Perform the operation,
$(5x^3 + 3x^2-4x + 2) + (-5x^2-3)$.

   A. $5x^3-2x^2-4x + 1$

   B. $5x^3-2x^2-4x-1$

   C. $5x^3 + 2x^2-4x-1$

   D. $5x^3 + 2x^2-4x + 1$

33. Simplify $\left(\frac{x^3y^{-2}}{x^{-2}y^3}\right)^5$.

   A. $\frac{1}{x^{25}y^{25}}$ C. $\frac{x^{25}}{y^{25}}$

   B. $\frac{y^{25}}{x^{25}}$ D. $x^{25}y^{25}$

34. Simplify $\left(\frac{xy^0}{z^2}\right)^2$.

   A. $\frac{x^2}{z^4y}$ C. $\frac{x^2}{z^4}$

   B. $\frac{x^2y}{z^4}$ D. x^2z^4

35. Simplify $((2^{-2})^{-1})^{-2}$.

   A. $\frac{1}{16}$ C. 8

   B. $\frac{1}{8}$ D. 16

36. Solve $x^3 = -8$.

   A. -4 C. 2

   B. -2 D. 4

37. The number 22 is what percent of 54?

   A. 22%   C. 41%

   B. 29%   D. 76%

38. How many dogs are necessary to make a cat-to-dog ratio of 3:2 in an area with 1,425 cats?

   A. 285   C. 2,138

   B. 950   D. 2,375

39. How many men does a company employ if it has 420 employees and 35% are women?

   A. 35   C. 273

   B. 147   D. 420

40. If a truck's initial speed is 60 mph and its final speed is 100 mph, what is its percent change in speed?

   A. 17%   C. 40%

   B. 33%   D. 67%

41. If a company's revenue changes from $123 million to $118 million in a month, how quickly is it increasing in a year?

   A. $-$$60 million   C. $5 million

   B. $-$$5 million   D. $60 million

42. A rectangular garden needs a border. The length is $15\frac{3}{5}$ feet, and the width is $3\frac{2}{3}$ feet. What is the perimeter in feet?

    A. $18\frac{5}{8}$ C. $37\frac{1}{4}$

    B. $19\frac{4}{15}$ D. $38\frac{8}{15}$

43. The level of a river during a flood was 39.45 feet. After a week, the water level declined to 18.97 feet. What was the amount of decrease in feet?

    A. 20.38   C. 21.38

    B. 20.48   D. 21.48

44. A piece of wood that is $5\frac{2}{3}$ feet long has $1\frac{1}{4}$ feet cut off. How many feet of wood remain?

    A. $4\frac{1}{12}$ C. $6\frac{1}{12}$

    B. $4\frac{5}{12}$ D. $6\frac{5}{12}$

45. Benjamin buys $3\frac{1}{3}, 2\frac{1}{2},$ and $1\frac{3}{4}$ of yards of fabric at a store. How many total yards did he purchase?

    A. $6\frac{5}{12}$ C. $7\frac{7}{12}$

    B. $6\frac{5}{9}$ D. $7\frac{7}{9}$

46. A small landscaping company mows lawns and has three 5.4-gallon gas cans. One day, the landscapers empty the gas cans three times. How many gallons of gas did they use?

    A. 10.8   C. 32.4

    B. 16.2   D. 48.6

47. Convert 0.5 kiloliter to milliliters.

    A. 50,000 milliliters

    B. 500,000 milliliters

    C. 5,000,000 milliliters

    D. 50,000,000 milliliters

48. Convert 750 millilitesrs to quarts.

    A. 0.0795 quarts

    B. 0.795 quarts

    C. 7.95 quarts

    D. 79.5 quarts

49. Convert 9 pints to liters.

    A. 4.25 liters

    B. 4.50 liters

    C. 8.49 liters

    D. 9.54 liters

50. Convert 18 miles to kilometers.

    A. 19.61 kilometers

    B. 28.98 kilometers

    C. 39.22 kilometers

    D. 57.96 kilometers

SECTION II. READING COMPREHENSION

You have 50 minutes to complete 47 questions.

Please read the text below and answer questions 1-3.

Publishers typically pay male authors slightly higher advances than female authors. They also price men's books higher, which results in higher royalty payments for male creators. Male authors are more likely than female authors to win literary awards, receive speaking invitations, and gain attention from major reviewers, all of which drive sales.

1. **Which phrase best describes the topic of the group of sentences in the paragraph?**

   A. An analysis of literary award winners

   B. Gender differences in author income

   C. A description of a book reviewer's day

   D. Resources for increasing author income

2. **Which of the following sentences would best function as a topic sentence to unite the information in the paragraph?**

   A. Gender differences in author pay primarily result from the fact that male authors appeal to a broader audience base.

   B. Although writers do not have fixed salaries, entrenched stereotyping results in a substantial pay gap between male and female authors.

   C. Authors can access a wide variety of income streams including fees for new work, royalties, speaking fees for public appearances, and more.

   D. Substantial evidence suggests that female authors simply do not produce work with the same impressive visionary quality as their greatest male peers.

3. **Which sentence provides another supporting detail to address the topic of the sentences in the paragraph?**

   A. Many young people dream of being famous writers, but authors face a difficult path to financial success with their work.

   B. Many female authors have recently come forward with alarming stories of sexual harassment and assault by powerful members of their industry.

   C. Very few contemporary authors are able to earn a living solely off their published works, so most rely on other sources of income to pay the bills.

   D. Numerous studies show that both publishers and readers are more likely to buy the same book if the author has a male name rather than a female name.

Read the following passage and answer questions 4-9.

Most people under age 35 spend too much time on social media. Statistics show that over nine out of ten teens go online using a mobile device daily, and seven out of ten use more than one major social media site. This is too much. Teens and young adults must limit their use of social media or face deteriorating relationships in real life. You know how frustrating it feels to try to talk to someone who constantly disengages to check a phone. Interacting online can be fun, but it never provides as much satisfaction as talking with actual human beings. Social media shouldn't be the primary social outlet for young people because people who rely mainly on

the Internet for social interaction are unhappy and unfulfilled.

4. **What is the primary argument in the passage?**

   A. All young people face emotional and social problems.

   B. Teens and young adults should limit their social media use.

   C. People under age 35 have never known life without the Internet.

   D. Disengaging to check a phone can damage real-life social interactions.

5. **Which excerpt from the text, if true, is a fact?**

   A. Most people under age 35 spend too much time on social media.

   B. Statistics show that over nine out of ten teens go online using a mobile device daily.

   C. Teens and young adults must limit their use of social media or face deteriorating relationships in real life.

   D. Interacting online can be fun, but it never provides as much satisfaction as talking with actual human beings.

6. Re-read the following sentence from the passage:

Teens and young adults must limit their use of social media or face deteriorating relationships in real life.

What type of faulty reasoning does this sentence display?

A. Either/or fallacy

B. Circular reasoning

C. Bandwagon argument

D. False statement of cause and effect

7. Re-read the following sentence from the passage:

Interacting online can be fun, but it never provides as much satisfaction as talking with actual human beings.

The reasoning in this sentence is faulty because it makes a(n):

A. circular statement.

B. overgeneralization.

C. bandwagon argument.

D. false statement of cause and effect.

8. Re-read the following sentence from the passage:

Social media shouldn't be the primary social outlet for young people because people who rely mainly on the Internet for social interaction are unhappy and unfulfilled.

The reasoning in this sentence is faulty because it:

A. suggests that an idea is good because everyone is doing it.

B. claims that there are only two ways to solve a complex problem.

C. restates the argument in different words instead of providing evidence.

D. assumes that people socialize because they want to feel happy and fulfilled.

9. Re-read the following sentence from the passage:

Most people under age 35 spend too much time on social media.

This sentence is an opinion because it:

A. reflects a belief, not a verifiable fact.

B. does not say how much is too much.

C. restricts its statement to people under 35.

D. lumps all people under 35 into one category.

Read the passages below and answer questions 10-18.

Electroconvulsive therapy was pioneered in the 1930s as a method for combatting severe psychiatric symptoms such as intractable depression and paranoid schizophrenia. This procedure, which involves delivering a deliberate electrical shock to the brain, was controversial from the beginning because it caused pain and short-term memory loss. It fell strongly out of public favor after the 1962 publication of Ken Kesey's novel *One Flew Over the Cuckoo's Nest*, which featured an unprincipled nurse using electroconvulsive therapy as a means of control over her patients. Paradoxically, medical advances at the time of the novel's publication made electroconvulsive therapy significantly safer and more humane.

Although the public is still generally opposed to electroconvulsive therapy, it remains a genuine option for psychiatric patients whose symptoms do not improve with medication. Medical professionals who offer this option should be especially careful to make clear distinctions between myth and reality. On this topic, unfortunately, many patients tend to rely on fiction rather than fact.

*

We were led into a stark exam room, where three doctors positioned themselves so Mama and I had no direct path to the door. The one in charge cleared his throat and told me my mother needed electroshock. My brain buzzed—almost as if it was hooked up to some crackpot brainwashing machine— as Big Doctor droned on about his

sadistic intentions. I didn't hear any of it. All I could think was that these people wanted to tie my mother down and stick wires in her ears.

When Big Doctor was finished, he flipped through the papers on his clipboard and asked if I had questions. I mumbled something noncommittal. Then, when he and his silent escort left, I grabbed Mama and beat it out of that wacko ward as fast as I could make her go.

10. **What is the purpose of the first paragraph of Passage 1?**
    A. To inform   C. To persuade
    B. To distract   D. To entertain

11. **What is the purpose of the second paragraph of Passage 1?**
    A. To inform   C. To persuade
    B. To distract   D. To entertain

12. **What is the primary purpose of Passage 2?**
    A. To inform   C. To persuade
    B. To distract   D. To entertain

13. **With which statement would the author of Passage 1 likely agree?**
    A. Patients who suffer from mental illness should sue Ken Kesey for libel.
    B. Electroconvulsive therapy is a ready solution for every psychiatric complaint.
    C. No twenty-first century patient should ever receive electroconvulsive therapy.
    D. Medical patients should try options such as medication before electroconvulsive therapy.

14. **Which detail from Passage 1 supports the conclusion that patients should try other options before electing to undergo electroconvulsive therapy?**

    A. This procedure...was controversial from the beginning because it caused pain and short-term memory loss.

    B. Ken Kesey's novel *One Flew Over the Cuckoo's Nest*...featured an unprincipled nurse using electroconvulsive therapy as a means of control over her patients.

    C. Electroconvulsive therapy...remains a genuine option for patients whose symptoms do not improve with medication.

    D. Paradoxically, medical advances at the time of the novel's publication made electroconvulsive therapy significantly safer and more humane.

15. **The author of Passage 1 would most likely criticize the author of Passage 2 for:**

    A. failing to listen to the doctor's explanations.

    B. making no attempt to protect her ailing mother.

    C. feeling threatened by her physical circumstances.

    D. asking too many questions and wasting the doctor's time.

16. **The author of Passage 1 would most likely criticize the doctor in Passage 2 for:**

    A. revealing medical information to the patient's family members.

    B. denying the patient and her family the chance to ask questions.

    C. taking control of the meeting instead of letting underlings speak.

    D. neglecting to anticipate the feelings of his patient and her family.

17. **Which details from Passage 2 suggest that the author has a negative outlook about medical professionals?**

    A. She describes feeling trapped in a room by doctors, one of whom she calls "sadistic."

    B. She describes feeling outnumbered when she makes reasoned arguments to a doctor she calls "wacko."

    C. She describes feeling bored by the idea that the doctor wants to "tie [her] mother down and stick wires in her ears."

    D. She describes feeling excited by the prospect of seeing her mother hooked up to a pseudo-medical "brainwashing machine."

18. **The author of Passage 1 supports her points primarily by:**

    A. telling humanizing stories.

    B. relying on facts and logic.

    C. pointing to expert sources.

    D. using fear tactics and manipulation.

Please read the text below and answer questions 19-23.

It is perhaps unsurprising that fad diets are so common given the level of obesity in American society. But over the long term, most fad diets are harmful both to the health and to the waistline. Many such diets advocate cutting out one major nutrient, such as fats or carbohydrates. Others suggest fasting over long periods or eating from fixed menu options that may not meet the body's needs. Most of these diets are highly impractical, and many lead directly or indirectly to binge eating and other unhealthy behaviors.

19. The topic of this paragraph is:

A. fasting.

B. obesity.

C. fad diets.

D. binge eating.

20. The topic sentence of this paragraph is:

A. But over the long term, most fad diets are harmful both to the health and to the waistline.

B. Many such diets advocate cutting out one major nutrient, such as fats or carbohydrates.

C. It is perhaps unsurprising that fad diets are so common given the level of obesity in American society.

D. Most of these diets are highly impractical, and many lead directly or indirectly to binge eating and other unhealthy behaviors.

21. If the author added a description of a man who attempted several fad diets and ended up heavier than ever, what type of information would this be?

A. A main idea

B. A topic sentence

C. A supporting detail

D. An off-topic sentence

22. Read the following description of the paragraph:

The author argues unfairly against fad diets without taking their good qualities into account.

Why is this *not* a valid description of the main idea?

A. It is not accurate; the author of the paragraph is stating facts, not opinions.

B. It is not objective; the person summarizing the main idea is adding a judgment.

C. It is not accurate; the author of the paragraph does not argue against fad diets.

D. It is not objective; the person summarizing the main idea ignores a sentence about the benefits of dieting.

23. Why doesn't a statistic about early childhood obesity rates belong in this paragraph?

   A. It does not directly support the main idea that fad diets are harmful.

   B. Readers might feel hopeless to solve the problem the author identifies.

   C. Statistics should never be used as supporting details in persuasive writing.

   D. It would act as a second topic sentence and confuse readers about the main idea.

Read the following passage and answer questions 24-27.

You know what I hate? Businesses that rely on contract workers and freelancers instead of regular employees.

Don't hit me with arguments about grater freedom for workers. Freedom isn't free if your bleeding out in the street.

Sound the alarm, people! Workers are suffering! No benefits means you're out of luck if you get sick and can't do your job. Plus, studies show freelancers don't make as much money as regular employees.

--From Rod's Job Blog at rodtalksaboutjobs.com

24. Which of the following is not a sign that the reader should be skeptical of this source?

   A. The passage contains typos and spelling errors.

   B. The author presents opinion information as if it is fact.

   C. There is no clear information about the author's credentials.

   D. The passage comes from a personal blog with a .com address.

25. Why should a reader be skeptical of the point about freelancers not making as much money as regular employees?

   A. The argument is not based in logic.

   B. Some freelancers make plenty of money.

   C. The source of the information is not clear.

   D. The sentence contains grammatical errors.

26. A reader should be skeptical of the line "Freedom isn't free if your (sic) bleeding out in the street" because it:

   A. appears to use objective language but is actually hiding gender bias.

   B. uses emotional language without responding to the opposing argument.

   C. seems to present an expert point of view but does not name the source.

   D. makes no attempt to defend regular workers in a discussion of the economy.

27. **A student is writing a paper on employment trends and wants to quote an expert's opinion. What type of site would provide the most credible alternative to Rod's Job Blog?**

    A. A different post on Rod's Jobs Blog

    B. A different blog with a .net address

    C. An opinion article by a recognized expert in the field

    D. A government website tracking employment statistics

Read the paragraph below and answer questions 28-32.

Until about 1850, few people living in temperate climates had ever had the opportunity to taste a banana. Only after the invention of the steamship could importers and exporters reliably transport this fruit to North America and Europe. Railways and refrigeration were two other vital components in the development of the banana trade. Today, bananas are a major export in several Central and South American countries as well as the Philippines. Around the world, people in climates that cannot support banana production now have access to plentiful inexpensive bananas.

28. **Which sentence provides an effective summary of the text above?**

    A. The author of this paragraph really likes bananas and researched them thoroughly.

    B. Shipping and refrigeration technology helped bananas become a major export crop.

    C. This paragraph should include more detail about the development of the banana trade.

    D. Before 1850, most Americans and Europeans had never had the opportunity to taste a banana.

29. **Read the following summary of the paragraph above.**

    According to John K. Miller, the invention of shipping and refrigeration technology helped bananas become a major export crop. The banana trade is an important source of income for many countries around the world, and consumers can buy bananas easily even in places where bananas do not grow.

    What makes this summary effective?

    A. It makes a judgment on the original text without being unfair.

    B. It restates the ideas of the original text in completely new words.

    C. It rearranges the ideas of the original text into a different sequence.

    D. It highlights ideas from the original text that were not stated explicitly.

30. **Which summary sentence retains language too close to the original text?**

   A. The author of this paragraph really likes bananas and researched them thoroughly.

   B. This paragraph should include more detail about the development of the banana trade.

   C. Before 1850, most Americans and Europeans had never had the opportunity to taste a banana.

   D. The technological developments of the Industrial Revolution helped create a global banana trade.

31. **Which summary sentence fails to be objective?**

   A. The author of this paragraph really likes bananas and researched them thoroughly.

   B. This paragraph should include more detail about the development of the banana trade.

   C. Before 1850, most Americans and Europeans had never had the opportunity to taste a banana.

   D. The technological developments of the Industrial Revolution helped create a global banana trade.

32. **Read the following sentence.**

   Nobody would eat bananas today if modern shipping and refrigeration technology had never been invented.

   Why doesn't this sentence belong in a summary of the paragraph above?

   A. It concerns supporting details and not main ideas.

   B. It adheres too closely to the original author's language.

   C. It fails to make a clear judgment about the original text.

   D. It does not accurately state an idea from the original text.

Read the passage and answer questions 33-36.

Dear Dr. Rodriguez,

I am writing to request that you change my daughter Amelia's chemistry grade. Amelia is a brilliant and capable girl who does not deserve an F in your class. Incidentally, I am sure you recall our family's substantial donation to your school district last year. I was led to believe we would no longer be troubled by petty grade issues or incompetent teachers after I wrote that check. In fact, I feel compelled to forward this message to your superiors to make certain the issue is dealt with promptly, and to ensure that we have no future misunderstandings.

Sincerely,

Violetta D. Johannsen

33. **Which adjective best describes the tone of this passage?**

   A. Friendly   C. Hopeless

   B. Arrogant   D. Respectful

34. **Which phrase from the passage has an openly hostile and superior tone?**

    A. I am writing to request

    B. brilliant and capable

    C. incompetent teachers

    D. to make certain

35. **What mood would this passage most likely evoke in the chemistry teacher, Dr. Rodriguez?**

    A. Fury   C. Calm

    B. Glee   D. Respect

36. **Which transition word or phrase from the passage adds emphasis to the writer's point?**

    A. And   C. In fact

    B. After   D. Incidentally

Read the passage below and answer questions 37-42.

The train was the most amazing thing ever even though it didn't go "choo choo." The toddler pounded on the railing of the bridge and supplied the sound herself. "Choo choo! Choo choooooo!" she shouted as the train cars whizzed along below.

In the excitement, she dropped her favorite binky.

Later, when she noticed the binky missing, all the joy went out of the world. The wailing could be heard three houses down. The toddler's usual favorite activities were garbage—even waving to Hank the garbage man, which she refused to do, so that Hank went away looking mildly hurt. It was clear the little

girl would never, ever, ever recover from her loss.

Afterward, she played at the park.

37. **Which adjectives best describe the tone of the passage?**

    A. Ironic, angry

    B. Earnest, angry

    C. Ironic, humorous

    D. Earnest, humorous

38. **Which sentence from the passage is clearly ironic?**

    A. "Choo choo! Choo choooooo!" she shouted as the train cars whizzed along below.

    B. Later, when she noticed the binky missing, all the joy went out of the world.

    C. The wailing could be heard three houses down.

    D. Afterward, she played at the park.

39. **The author of the passage first establishes the ironic tone by:**

    A. describing the child's trip to play at the park.

    B. calling the train "the most amazing thing ever."

    C. pretending that the child can make the sounds "choo choooo!"

    D. claiming inaccurately that the lost binky was the child's "favorite."

40. **Reread the following sentence:**

It was clear the little girl would never, ever, ever recover from her loss.

Which adjective could describe an effective reader's mood when reading this line in the context of the passage?

A. Amused

C. Horrified

B. Worried

D. Jubilant

41. **Which word or phrase does *not* function as a transition in the passage?**

A. Later

C. Afterward

B. Below

D. In the excitement

42. **The transitions "later" and "afterward" link ideas in the passage by showing:**

A. when events happen in time.

B. how certain ideas contrast.

C. examples that illustrate ideas.

D. cause-and-effect relationships.

Read the following passages and answer questions 43-47.

As a parent, I find television and movie rating systems unhelpful. Ratings systems are not human. Their scores are based on numbers: how many bad words, how many gory scenes. To me, that makes no sense. Nobody else knows my kids like I do, so nobody else can say what's okay for them to watch.

In my experience, the content a government organization rates as PG or PG-13 may or may not be appropriate for my 9-, 14-, and 16-year-olds. My youngest is quite mature for his age, and I'm fine with him hearing a bad word or two as a part of a meaningful story.

Violence concerns me more. I won't let even my 16-year-old watch frivolous violence or horror. But I don't shelter him from realistic violence. My little guy still has to stay out of the room for the bloody stuff. But eventually, kids need to know what's out there.

43. **The primary purpose of this passage is to:**

A. decide

C. persuade

B. inform

D. entertain

44. **The author of this passage would be most likely to agree that:**

A. kids should not watch television or movies at all until they are in their teens.

B. government rating systems should have more levels to make them more useful.

C. it is never appropriate to prevent any human being from watching any show or movie.

D. another parent should have the right to let her own kids watch extremely violent movies.

45. **The author of this passage would be likely to support an effort to:**

    A. create a government system to recommend ages for reading children's books.

    B. prevent kids from attending movies in the theater without their parents' presence.

    C. provide parents more information about the content of children's shows and movies.

    D. change the age for watching PG-13 movies down to 10 because today's kids are more savvy.

46. **What is the most likely reason for the author's decision to include the phrase "as a parent" at the beginning?**

    A. This phrase provides a reason to support her opinion.

    B. She is implying that non-parents cannot know what kids need.

    C. This phrase provides a transition from the points she made earlier.

    D. She is establishing herself as a knowledgeable source on this topic.

47. **When the author says ratings systems are "based on numbers," she is developing the point that:**

    A. logic and reasoning have no place in parenting.

    B. the only numbers that matter are her children's ages.

    C. some decisions should be made on a case-by-case basis.

    D. she is not good enough at math to rely on ratings systems.

SECTION III. VOCABULARY & GENERAL KNOWLEDGE

You have 50 minutes to complete 50 questions.

1. Which of the following suffixes means **act, process**?

   A. -able C. -less

   B. -tion D. -ible

2. Which of the following suffixes means **happened in the past**?

   A. -an C. -en

   B. -ed D. -er

3. Which of the following suffixes means **the study of**?

   A. -less C. -ition

   B. -able D. -logy

4. Which of the following root words means **to throw**?

   A. ject C. rupt

   B. dict D. mort

5. Which of the following root words means **to build**?

   A. sect C. sol

   B. script D. struct

6. Which of the following prefixes means **water**?

   A. auto- C. hydro-

   B. con- D. post-

7. What is the best definition of the word **multifaceted**?

   A. Having one side

   B. Having two sides

   C. Having many sides

   D. Having no sides

8. What is the best definition of the word **dissect**?

   A. To combine into one piece

   B. To separate into pieces

   C. To organize multiple pieces

   D. To move around different pieces

9. The use of the suffix *-ous* in the word *parsimonious* indicates what about a person?

   A. He/she is full of stinginess

   B. He/she is against stinginess

   C. He/she is supportive of stinginess

   D. He/she is a person who studies stinginess

10. Which of the following prefixes means **incorrect**?

    A. un- C. mis-

    B. non- D. over-

11. What is the best definition of the word **pugnacious**?

    A. Rude C. Deceiving

    B. Harmful D. Combative

12. The use of the prefix *sub-* in the word *subservient* indicates that a person is which of the following?

    A. Equal with someone else

    B. Better than someone else

    C. In charge of someone else

    D. Obedient to someone else

13. What is the best definition of the word <u>rupture</u>?

    A. To seep   C. To swell

    B. To heal   D. To burst

14. Which of the following prefixes means <u>between</u>?

    A. sub-   C. inter-

    B. anti-   D. trans-

15. The use of the prefix *pre-* in the word *premonition* indicates which the following?

    A. Something good has happened

    B. Something is known before it happens

    C. Something does not have a chance of happening

    D. Something will happen as a result of something else

16. Which of the following prefixes means <u>self</u>?

    A. con-   C. auto-

    B. man-   D. post-

17. Select the meaning of the underlined word in the sentence.

    The teacher listened to the student's excuse with an <u>incredulous</u> smile.

    A. Forced   C. Insincere

    B. Amused   D. Disbelieving

18. The use of the prefix *re-* in the word *reinstate* indicates which of the following about a person's position?

    A. It has been restored

    B. It has been revealed

    C. It has been removed

    D. It has been relocated

19. What is the best definition of the word <u>translucent</u>?

    A. Blocking all light

    B. Blinding with light

    C. Giving off colorful light

    D. Letting some light through

20. What is the best definition of the word <u>miscreant</u>?

    A. Careless   C. Villainous

    B. Uninformed   D. Opinionated

21. What is the best definition of the word <u>veritable</u>?

    A. Noble   C. Forceful

    B. Genuine   D. Exaggerated

22. Which of the following prefixes means <u>with</u>?

    A. bio-   C. con-

    B. per-   D. trans-

23. Which of the following root words means <u>color</u>?

    A. vid   C. chrom

    B. chron   D. therm

24. Select the context clue from the following sentence that helps you define the multiple meaning word <u>hatch</u>.

    The group met each month to <u>hatch</u> a plan to overthrow the government.

    A. "group"   C. "plan"

    B. "met"   D. "overthrow"

25. Select the context clue from the following sentence that helps you define the multiple meaning word <u>operation</u>.

The family has always worked together to run their small farming <u>operation</u>.

A. "family" C. "worked"

B. "always" D. "farming"

26. Select the correct definition of the underlined word having multiple meanings in the sentence.

Natalie's fingers were calloused after practicing her <u>bass</u>.

A. Kind of fish

B. Low and deep sound

C. Lowest male singing voice

D. A guitar with four strings that makes low sounds

27. Select the correct definition of the underlined word that has multiple meanings in the sentence.

When the young boy saw his angry mother coming toward him, he made a <u>bolt</u> for the door.

A. A large roll of cloth

B. A quick movement in a particular direction

C. A sliding bar that is used to lock a window or door

D. A bright line of light appearing in the sky during a storm

28. Select the context clue from the following sentence that helps you define the word <u>unkempt</u>.

Our neighbors across the street have an <u>unkempt</u> front lawn with lawn furniture and knickknacks strewn in every corner.

A. "across the street"

B. "front lawn"

C. "knickknacks strewn"

D. "every corner"

29. Select the correct definition of the underlined word that has more than one meaning in the sentence.

Good thing the lamp has a heavy <u>base</u> or it would have fallen when Henry bumped into it.

A. The bottom or lowest part of something

B. The places a runner must touch in baseball

C. The place where people in the military live and work

D. The main ingredient to which other things are added

30. Select the context clue from the following sentence that helps you define the word <u>facetious</u>.

It was clear that Timothy was being <u>facetious</u> since he smirked after saying he was willing to help.

A. "clear"   C. "saying "

B. "smirked"   D. "help"

31. Select the correct definition of the underlined word that has multiple meanings in the sentence.

    It is not legal to <u>harbor</u> an escaped convict in your home.

    A. To hide someone

    B. To contain something

    C. To keep a feeling inside

    D. To have a thought in one's mind

32. Select the context clue from the following sentence that helps you define the word <u>emulate</u>.

    Felicia always tried to <u>emulate</u> her big sister, so she would often imitate the way she spoke, moved, and how she dressed.

    A. "tried"   C. "imitate "

    B. "often"   D. "way"

33. Select the context clue from the following sentence that helps you define the word <u>reconnaissance</u>.

    Several helicopters were sent out to conduct a <u>reconnaissance</u> of the enemy.

    A. "several"   C. "conduct"

    B. "helicopters"   D. "enemy"

34. Select the correct definition of the underlined word that has more than one meaning in the sentence.

    The teacher informed the student that the final <u>draft</u> of her report was due by the end of the week.

    A. The cool air moving in a closed space

    B. A version of a document such as a written paper

    C. The system by which professional sports teams choose players

    D. An order for the payment of money from one entity to another

35. Select the correct definition of the underlined word that has multiple meanings in the sentence.

    Sandra needed to <u>crop</u> the photograph to make it fit into the frame.

    A. To cut off a part of

    B. To bite off and eat the tops of

    C. To produce or make a plant grow

    D. To come on or appear unexpectedly

36. Select the context clue from the following sentence that helps you define the word <u>pungent</u>.

    The <u>pungent</u> odor in the room made everyone's eyes tear for a few minutes.

    A. "odor"   C. "made"

    B. "room"   D. "tear"

37. Select the context clue from the following sentence that helps you define the multiple meaning word <u>program</u>.

    This morning I watched a <u>program</u> about the easiest brunch recipes to make.

    A. "morning"   C. "brunch"

    B. "watched"   D. "make"

38. Adding which of the following to prefixes to <u>thyroid</u> would describe the area next to the thyroid?

    A. Sub-   C. Para-

    B. Peri-   D. Super-

39. Based on your knowledge of medical roots, prefixes, and suffixes, which of the following words means a disease of the muscle or muscle tissue?

    A. Myopathy

    B. Osteopathy

    C. Enteropathy

    D. Encephalopathy

40. Based on your knowledge of medical roots, prefixes, and suffixes, which of the following words means the study of the nervous system?

    A. Radiology   C. Cardiology

    B. Neurology   D. Dermatology

41. Read the following sentence.

The doctor was treating the patient for gastric pain.

What kind of pain was the patient experiencing?

    A. Chest pain   C. Stomach pain

    B. Throat pain   D. Lower back pain

42. Based on your knowledge of medical roots, prefixes, and suffixes, which of the following words means the study of the structure and function of cells?

    A. Cytology

    B. Endocrinology

    C. Rheumatology

    D. Gastroenterology

43. Select the meaning of the underlined word in the sentence.

The doctor performed a <u>nephrectomy</u> on the patient.

    A. Viewing of the patient's liver

    B. Removal of the patient's kidney

    C. Puncture of the patient's tumor

    D. Surgical repair of the patient's lung

44. Read the following sentence.

The nurse's instructed the patient to take her <u>ocular</u> medication twice daily.

What kind of medicine is the patient taking?

    A. Eye medicine

    B. Joint medicine

    C. Stomach medicine

    D. Blood pressure medicine

45. Read the following sentence.

The patient was <u>hemotoxic</u> and had to be treated immediately.

What kind of condition is the patient suffering from?

    A. Heart pains

    B. Liver failure

    C. Blood poisoning

    D. Tissue hardening

46. Based on your knowledge of roots, prefixes, and suffixes what does <u>epidermis</u> mean?

    A. The inner layer of tissue

    B. The outer layer of the skin

    C. The area under the muscles

    D. The area around the spinal cord

47. In this sentence the suffix indicates that the doctor plans to do an excision on which body part?

    The doctor needs to perform a pneumonectomy on the patient.

    A. Lung   C. Heart

    B. Liver   D. Kidney

48. Select the meaning of the underlined word in the sentence.

    The doctor performed an endoscopy on the patient.

    A. Examination of the patient's throat

    B. Viewing of the patient's internal parts

    C. Surgical removal of the patient's spleen

    D. Artificial opening of the patient's abdomen

49. In this sentence the root indicates that the patient has inflammation of which body part?

    The patient was suffering from hepatitis.

    A. Liver   C. Spleen

    B. Kidney   D. Gallbladder

50. Select the meaning of the underlined word in the sentence.

    The scientists were studying human osteocytes to learn more about them.

    A. Bone cells

    B. Organ tumors

    C. Tissue diseases

    D. Nerve abnormalities

Section IV. Grammar

You have 50 minutes to complete 50 questions.

1. **What is the correct plural of** *bush*?

   A. Bush   C. Bushes

   B. Bushs   D. Bushies

2. **What is the correct plural of** *century*?

   A. Centurys   C. Centuries

   B. Centures   D. Centuryies

3. **We saw a _____ in the woods while hiking.**

   A. bair   C. bare

   B. baer   D. bear

4. **We _____ the newspaper every day.**

   A. red   C. reed

   B. reid   D. read

5. **Fill in the blank with the correctly capitalized form.**

   My favorite book in the Harry Potter series is _____.

   A. *harry potter and the prisoner of azkaban*

   B. *Harry Potter and the prisoner of azkaban*

   C. *Harry Potter And The Prisoner Of Azkaban*

   D. *Harry Potter and the Prisoner of Azkaban*

6. **Fill in the blank with the correctly capitalized form.**

   _____ is part of the United Kingdom.

   A. northern ireland

   B. Northern Ireland

   C. Northern ireland

   D. northern Ireland

7. **Fill in the blank with the correctly capitalized form.**

   Everyone wants to live in _____ _____, because it has nice weather and beaches.

   A. southern California

   B. Southern California

   C. Southern california

   D. southern california

8. **Fill in the blank with the correctly capitalized form.**

   In the 2018 Super Bowl, the _____ played against the _____.

   A. philadelphia eagles, new england patriots

   B. Philadelphia eagles, New England patriots

   C. Philadelphia Eagles, New England Patriots

   D. Philadelphia Eagles, new england Patriots

9. **What is the mistake in the following sentence?**

   The highestranking officer can choose his own work, including his own hours.

   A. *Highestranking* needs a hyphen.

   B. There should be a comma after *officer*.

   C. There should be no comma after *work*.

   D. There should be a semicolon after *work*.

10. **What is the mistake in the following sentence?**

    The video game was intense; I needed state of the art weapons and armor to slay a dragon.

    A. The semicolon is misplaced.

    B. *Video game* should be hyphenated.

    C. *State of the art* should be hyphenated.

    D. There should be a comma between *weapons* and *and*.

11. **What is the mistake in the following sentence?**

    Queen Elizabeths grandsons are both married to smart, beautiful, and kind women.

    A. *Elizabeths* needs an apostrophe.

    B. *Grandsons* needs an apostrophe.

    C. There should be a colon after *to*.

    D. There should be a comma after *kind*.

12. **What is the mistake in the following sentence?**

    It's unfortunately raining outside today.

    A. *It's* does not need an apostrophe.

    B. There should be a comma after *outside*.

    C. There should be a period after *unfortunately*.

    D. There should be commas before and after *unfortunately*.

13. **Select the correct nouns for the blanks in the following sentence.**

    We can use these _____ to cut these fillets of _____.

    A. knives, salmon

    B. knifes, salmon

    C. knifes, salmons

    D. knives, salmons

14. **Select the sentence that has a noun as its subject.**

    A. Whose turn is it?

    B. Susan made dinner.

    C. I walked to the bus stop.

    D. They didn't know the answer.

15. **Select the correct words to complete the following sentence.**

    I have _____ due tomorrow.

    A. many homework

    B. many homeworks

    C. a lot of homework

    D. a lot of homeworks

16. **Select the sentence that contains three nouns.**

    A. Try not to slip on the ice.

    B. Weddings are joyous occasions.

    C. Ivana, Helen, and Tony left early.

    D. Hitoshi will visit us in San Francisco.

17. Select the noun to which the underlined pronoun refers.

Greta Garbo, who performed in both silent and talking pictures, is my favorite actress.

A. actress

B. pictures

C. performed

D. Greta Garbo

18. Select the noun to which the underlined pronoun refers.

Leon and Josiah took their entrance exams on Saturday, and I took mine on Sunday.

A. Me

B. exams

C. Sunday

D. entrance

19. Select the noun to which the underlined pronoun refers.

The fishermen caught three fish and fried them over the fire.

A. fire

B. fish

C. three

D. fishermen

20. Select the noun that the underlined adjectives describe.

Two weeks after his surgery, Henry felt strong and healthy.

A. weeks

B. his

C. surgery

D. Henry

21. Select the part of speech of the underlined word in the following sentence.

He hit the ball so hard that he was sure it was a home run!

A. Verb

B. Adverb

C. Adjective

D. Pronoun

22. Select the part of speech of the underlined word in the following sentence.

I thought the homework was very difficult.

A. Noun

B. Adverb

C. Adjective

D. Preposition

23. Select the musical title that contains an adverb.

A. *Follies*

B. *West Side Story*

C. *Into the Woods*

D. *Merrily We Roll Along*

24. Select the book title that does not contain a preposition.

A. *The Man in the Brown Suit*

B. *The Secret of Chimneys*

C. *Murder on the Orient Express*

D. *And Then There Were None*

25. Select another conjunction with the same meaning as the underlined conjunction.

History is my favorite subject, but I did not do well on the test.

A. so

B. since

C. yet

D. if

26. Select the book title that contains a conjunction.

A. *The Catcher in the Rye*

B. *Nine Stories*

C. *Franny and Zooey*

D. *A Perfect Day for Bananafish*

27. **Select the pair of correlative conjunctions that best completes the following sentence.**

    We can meet ____ at your office ____ at the station.

    A. either/or   C. as/as

    B. whether/or   D. both/but

28. **Select the response that correctly describes both of the underlined verbs.**

    When a buyer offered 5% below our asking price, our realtor advised us to accept the offer.

    A. Helping verbs

    B. Past tense verbs

    C. Present tense verbs

    D. Progressive tense verbs

29. **Select the helping verb that completes the following sentence.**

    Millions of people watched the news story on TV as it ____ unfolding.

    A. is   C. was

    B. did   D. would

30. **Select the sentence that best describes something that happens regularly.**

    A. Mary got up at 7:00.

    B. Mary gets up at 7:00.

    C. Mary is getting up at 7:00.

    D. Mary was getting up at 7:00.

31. **Select the correct verbs to complete the following sentence.**

    My dentist, who I ____ visited for years, ____ suddenly disappeared.

    A. has, has   C. has, have

    B. have, has   D. have, have

32. **Select the correct verbs to complete the following sentence.**

    As soon as the ship sets sail, the meteorologist ____ that a hurricane ____ coming.

    A. announce, is

    B. announce, are

    C. announces, is

    D. announces, are

33. **Select the correct verb to complete the following sentence.**

    The news I got ____ not the news I was expecting.

    A. are   C. were

    B. was   D. being

34. **Select the correct verb to complete the following sentence.**

    This box of toys ____ to be put away.

    A. ned   C. needs

    B. need   D. needing

35. **Which of the following options correctly fixes the fragment below?**

    After going to the movies.

    A. After going to dinner we went to the movies.

    B. After going to dinner we, went to the movies.

    C. After going to dinner, we went to the movies.

    D. After going to dinner, and we went to the movies.

36. **Which of the following is an example of a compound sentence?**

    A. Felix has taken Taekwondo for years, now he is a black belt.

    B. Felix has taken Taekwondo for years and now he is a black belt.

    C. Felix has taken Taekwondo for years, and now he is a black belt.

    D. Felix has taken Taekwondo for years because now he is a black belt.

37. **Which of the following is an example of a compound sentence?**

    A. Monte cannot run in the race tomorrow, he injured his ankle.

    B. Monte injured his ankle and cannot run in the race tomorrow.

    C. Monte injured his ankle, so he cannot run in the race tomorrow.

    D. Monte cannot run in the race tomorrow since he injured his ankle.

38. **Which of the following is an example of a complex sentence?**

    A. Timothy got a massage after running.

    B. After running, Timothy got a massage.

    C. Since Timothy went running he got a massage.

    D. Timothy went running, and then he got a massage.

39. **Fill in the blank with the correct subordinating conjunction.**

    You cannot go to the movies with your friends _____ you finish your homework.

    A. if   C. since

    B. once   D. unless

40. **Fill in the blank with the correct subordinating conjunction.**

    I had a bad stomach flu but started to regain my appetite, _____ is good news.

    A. so   C. which

    B. that   D. whereas

41. **Fill in the blank with the correct subordinating conjunction.**

    We will throw a pizza party _____ you win the game.

    A. if   C. since

    B. that   D. because

42. **Fill in the blank with the correct subordinating conjunction.**

    _____ the class was difficult, Allison passed with flying colors.

    A. If   C. Because

    B. Since   D. Although

43. **Identify the likely misplaced modifier in the following sentence.**

    The man in blue wore a large, gaudy hat on his head, which was ugly.

    A. in blue   C. gaudy

    B. large   D. which was ugly

44. **Which ending does not create a sentence with a dangling modifier?**

    After eating, _____.

    A. we watched the storm.

    B. the storm came.

    C. it rained.

    D. the weather turned bad.

45. **What type of error can be found in the following sentence?**

    Spinning their webs, I saw two spiders.

    A. Sentence fragment

    B. Misplaced modifier

    C. Incorrect verb tense

    D. Spelling error

46. **What type of error can be found in the following sentence?**

    The report earned an A that I wrote on the Korean War.

    A. Run-on sentence

    B. Incorrect subject-verb agreement

    C. Misplaced modifier

    D. Pronoun error

47. **Identify the direct object of the underlined verb in the following sentence.**

    Tommy <u>watched</u> a movie with Mary.

    A. Tommy

    B. watched

    C. a movie

    D. with Mary

48. **Identify the indirect object in the following sentence, if there is one.**

    Snowflakes fell softly to the ground.

    A. Snowflakes

    B. softly

    C. ground

    D. There is no indirect object.

49. **Identify the direct object in the following sentence.**

    William's sister painted a portrait for him.

    A. William's

    B. sister

    C. portrait

    D. him

50. **Identify the indirect object in the following sentence, if there is one.**

    When I go, I'll take you with me.

    A. you

    B. with

    C. me

    D. There is no indirect object.

SECTION V. BIOLOGY

You have 25 minutes to complete 25 questions.

1. **When using the scientific method, what does a researcher do immediately after proposing a scientific question?**
   A. Perform background research on the topic
   B. Analyze data to observe trends or patterns
   C. Collect information or data during an experiment
   D. Communicate results in an article or presentation

2. **Fats and steroids belong to what biomolecule class?**
   A. Lipids
   B. Proteins
   C. Nucleic acids
   D. Carbohydrates

3. **What is a benefit of a taxonomic system?**
   A. Researchers can describe how living things behave.
   B. Researchers can develop names for new organisms.
   C. Living things can be distinguished from nonliving things.
   D. Living things can be classified based on their molecular traits.

4. **What is a control variable?**
   A. The variable that is used for comparisons
   B. The responding variable in an experiment
   C. The manipulated variable in an experiment
   D. The variable that is measured or able to be changed

5. **Why is glycolysis a catabolic pathway?**
   A. Electrons are transferred from one molecule to another.
   B. Energy is released as glucose splits into pyruvate molecules.
   C. Several different types of molecules are formed as products.
   D. Different biomolecules used during this process are reduced.

6. **What happens during anabolic metabolism?**
   A. Energy is released.
   B. Energy is absorbed.
   C. Nutrients are recycled.
   D. Substances are broken down.

7. **What is the most basic unit of structure in living things?**
   A. Cell
   B. Organelle
   C. Oxygen
   D. Pigment

8. **Which statement is most strongly supported by the cell theory?**
   A. Plant cells have similar cell parts to animal cells.
   B. Cells house their genetic information in the nucleus.
   C. Blood cells arise from stem cells in the bone marrow.
   D. Nonliving things lack a cell and associated organelles.

9. A cell processes the conversion of carbohydrates to ATP to help perform various biological functions. Where does this conversion occur in the cell?

   A. Vacuole
   B. Lysosome
   C. Mitochondria
   D. Golgi apparatus

10. What is the basis for classifying an organism as either an autotroph or a heterotroph?

    A. The way an organism obtains its energy
    B. The organism's ranking in the taxonomic system
    C. The type of ecosystem in which an organism lives
    D. Whether the organism is unicellular or multicellular

11. What organelle is only associated with plant cells?

    A. Cell wall
    B. Ribosome
    C. Cytoplasm
    D. Golgi apparatus

12. What is the function of a lysosome?

    A. Store energy for future use
    B. Process genetic information
    C. Synthesize and package proteins
    D. Break down foods and old organelles

13. How many net ATP molecules are generated by the process of glycolysis?

    A. 2
    B. 6
    C. 32
    D. 34

14. During which phase of meiosis do chiasmata structures form?

    A. Prophase I
    B. Prophase II
    C. Metaphase I
    D. Metaphase II

15. Which statement correctly compares cytokinesis in plants and animals?

    A. Cytokinesis in plants involves a new cell wall, but it involves physically deforming the cell in animals.
    B. Cytokinesis in plants relies on formation of microtubules between the new cells, but actin plays this role in animals.
    C. Cytokinesis does not happen in plants, leading to multinucleate plant cells, but it involves forming a cell wall in animals.
    D. Cytokinesis in plants uses a line of mitochondria to separate the two new cells, but the endoplasmic reticulum is used in animals.

16. During which phase of the cell cycle is DNA copied?

    A. Mitotic
    B. First Gap
    C. Synthesis
    D. Second Gap

17. What molecule plays a direct role in chemiosmosis?

    A. glucose
    B. NADH
    C. O_2
    D. pyruvate

18. When would a cell most likely contain the most nucleotides?

    A. S
    B. G_1
    C. M
    D. G_2

19. If an organism has a total of 12 chromosomes, 12 is the _____ number of chromosomes.

    A. diploid
    C. haploid

    B. equivalent
    D. neutral

20. In DNA replication, a DNA strand is separated, and a

    A. complementary strand attaches.

    B. complementary strand is assembled.

    C. complementary strand replicates itself.

    D. complementary strand forms a double helix.

21. What would be the probability of a short pea plant (ss) and a tall pea plant (Ss) producing a heterozygous tall pea plant?

    A. 25%
    C. 75%

    B. 50%
    D. 100%

22. Once RNA polymerase reaches a stop codon on the DNA molecule, the enzyme detaches from the DNA and releases the RNA molecule

    A. into the cell for the next stage.

    B. into the cytoplasm for translation.

    C. into the nucleus for the next stage.

    D. into the cytoplasm for transcription.

23. Which statement best represents Mendel's experiments with garden peas?

    A. As a result, Mendel developed several theories that have since been disproved.

    B. Mendel realized he was on an incorrect track, which led him to other experimental media.

    C. As a result, Mendel developed foundational conclusions that are still valued and followed today.

    D. Mendel collaborated with others interested in genetics to develop heredity guidelines we still use today.

24. In genetics, Punnett squares are used to predict crosses between traits. What is the name of the factor that is used to signify each trait passed down from the parents of the offspring?

    A. Allele
    C. Chromosome

    B. Chromatid
    D. Enzyme

25. In eukaryotes, what does transcription produce?

    A. mRNA
    C. rRNA

    B. pre-mRNA
    D. tRNA

SECTION VI. CHEMISTRY

You have 25 minutes to complete 25 questions.

1. Why is the metric system used in science?

   A. The base units are used interchangeably.

   B. It is easy to remember how the system works.

   C. The units are expressed as a base of a hundred.

   D. It is a universally accepted way to report values.

2. Which part of the scientific method requires a researcher to create variables?

   A. Writing a procedure

   B. Testing a hypothesis

   C. Drafting a conclusion

   D. Formulating a hypothesis

3. Which analysis describes the results shown in the following image?

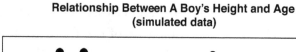

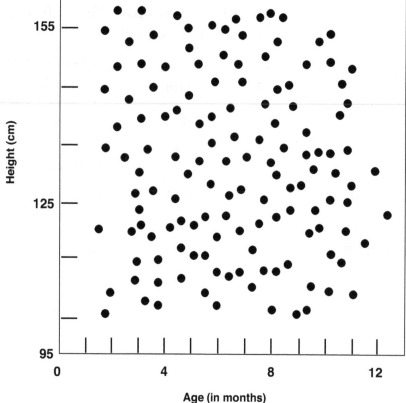

   A. As a baby gets older, he gets taller.

   B. Birth month is independent of height.

   C. Older boys are taller than younger boys

   D. A baby's height stays the same every month.

4. Based on the following graph, what does this data show?

Plot of weight by height

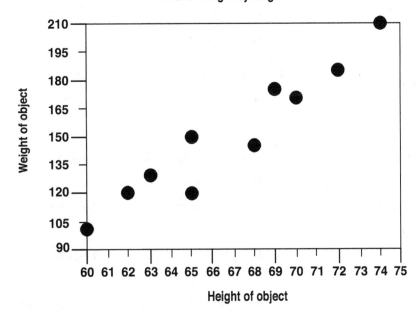

A. Weight is independent of height.

B. As height increases, weight also increases.

C. Weight is indirectly correlated with height.

D. A negative variation exists between weight and height.

5. Zinc-64 is one possible isotope of the element zinc. Which of the atoms described below is a different isotope of zinc?

A. 34 protons, 34 neutrons, 34 electrons

B. 34 protons, 30 neutrons, 34 electrons

C. 30 protons, 36 neutrons, 30 electrons

D. 64 protons, 34 neutrons, 34 electrons

6. Which of the following parts of an atom has the largest mass?

A. A proton

B. A neutron

C. The nucleus

D. The electron cloud

7. An electron has a mass of 9.11×10^{-31} kg. When this value is represented in standard notation, how many zeros are between the decimal point and the nearest non-zero digit?

A. 29

B. 30

C. 31

D. 32

8. A nanometer is equal to 1×10^{-9} meter. How is this value written in standard notation?

A. 0.0000000001 m

B. 0.000000001 m

C. 1,000,000,000 m

D. 10,000,000,000 m

9. The ratio of the mass of a proton to the mass of an electron is 1,840. How is this number represented in scientific notation?

    A. 0.184×10^4 C. 18.4×10^2

    B. 1.84×10^3 D. 184×10^1

10. A researcher is looking at a procedure that says he needs 0.0505 g of sodium. What unit of measurement does this describe?

    A. Length   C. Volume

    B. Time   D. Mass

11. What conversion formula is used to convert Celsius to Fahrenheit?

    A. $C = (\frac{9}{5})F + 32$

    B. $C = (\frac{5}{9})F + 32$

    C. $C = \frac{5}{9}(F - 32)$

    D. $C = \frac{9}{5}(F + 32)$

12. One microgram of medicine corresponds to how many grams?

    A. 0.000001   C. 0.0001

    B. 0.00001   D. 0.001

13. What is the Fahrenheit value for 110°C?

    A. 61   C. 198

    B. 78   D. 230

14. Which of the following describes a sample that is boiling?

    A. The energy of the particles is increasing.

    B. The particles are getting closer together.

    C. The temperature of the substance is increasing.

    D. The cohesive forces between particles are getting stronger.

15. At which temperature are all three halogens in the same state of matter?

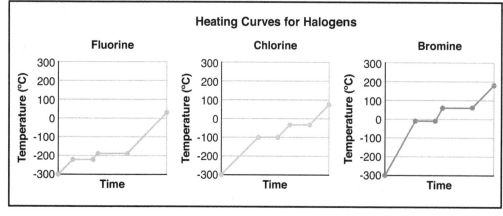

Heating Curves for Halogens

    A. -100°C   C. 10°C

    B. -10°C   D. 100°C

16. A good illustration to differentiate between the two types of properties is that mass and volume are _____ properties, but their ratio (density) is a(n) _____ property of matter.

   A. chemical, physical

   B. physical, chemical

   C. extensive, intensive

   D. intensive, extensive

17. Net water movement through a membrane in response to the concentration of a solute is called _____.

   A. bonding   C. osmosis

   B. diffusion   D. polarity

18. Which would turn litmus paper blue?

   A. HF   C. HNO_3

   B. KOH   D. $C_3H_6O_3$

19. Inside a plant, water has to travel up, against gravity, to reach all the leaves. What property does this illustrate?

   A. Adhesion   C. Cohesion

   B. Bonding   D. Polarity

20. If barium metal (Ba) and aluminum chloride ($AlCl_3$) react in a single-replacement reaction, what product(s) form?

   A. $BaAlCl_3$ C. $Al + BaCl_2$

   B. $AlBaCl_3$ D. $AlCl_3 + Ba$

21. If sodium sulfide (Na_2S) and hydrochloric acid (HCl) react in a double-replacement reaction, what product(s) form?

   A. Na_2SHCl C. $NaCl + H_2S$

   B. $NaHCl + S$ D. $HCl + Na_2S$

22. In the compound silicon tetrachloride ($SiCl_4$) shown below, how is silicon stable?

Silicon Tetrachloride
$SiCl_4$

Phosphorus Trichloride
PCl_3

Oxygen Dichloride
OCl_2

Chlorine Molecule
Cl_2

   A. Silicon shares a total of four electrons.

   B. Silicon shares a total of eight electrons.

   C. Silicon gives eight electrons to surrounding chlorine atoms.

   D. Silicon removes four electrons from surrounding chlorine atoms.

23. According to the Lewis structure below, what is the formula for methanol?

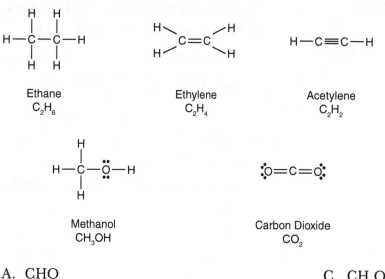

A. CHO

B. CH_3O

C. CH_4O

D. C_3HO

24. If 30 grams of $KClO_3$ is added to 100 grams of water at 0°C, some of the solute remains undissolved. What is the minimum temperature that must be attained to dissolve all the solute?

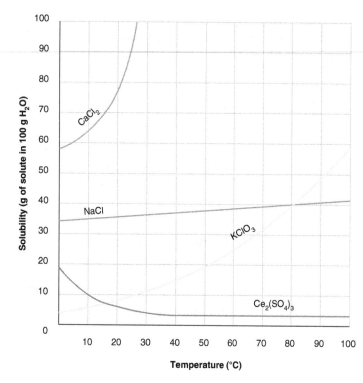

A. 30°C

B. 70°C

C. 80°C

D. 100°C

25. Using the following image, what substance is most likely a weak acid?

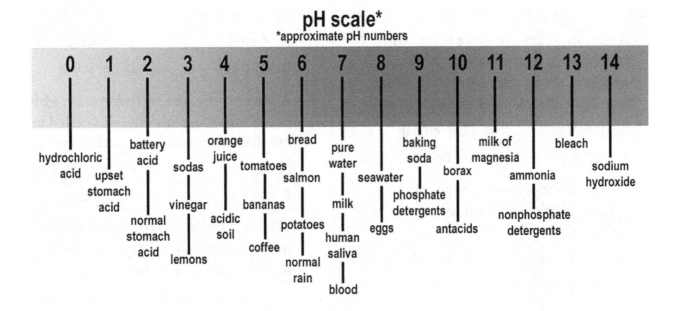

A. Antacid

B. Borax

C. Milk

D. Salmon

SECTION VII. ANATOMY & PHYSIOLOGY

You have 25 minutes to complete 25 questions.

1. A person wakes up with a fever. The body begins its response to locate the origin of the problem and fix it. What type of feedback mechanism is this?

    A. Equal
    C. Neutral
    B. Negative
    D. Positive

2. Which of the following types of tissues include cells of the immune system and of the blood?

    A. Connective
    C. Muscle
    B. Epithelial
    D. Neural

3. Which valve regulates blood flow between the right atrium and right ventricle?

    A. Aortic
    C. Pulmonary
    B. Mitral
    D. Tricuspid

4. Which is the correct order of formed elements in blood from smallest to largest cell size?

    A. Erythrocytes, thrombocytes, and leukocytes
    B. Thrombocytes, leukocytes, and erythrocytes
    C. Thrombocytes, erythrocytes, and leukocytes
    D. Leukocytes, erythrocytes, and thrombocytes

5. Which organ branches off into the bronchi?

    A. Alveolus
    C. Nose
    B. Larynx
    D. Trachea

6. Where are the vocal cords located?

    A. Capillary
    C. Nose
    B. Larynx
    D. Trachea

7. After a person eats birthday cake, which of the following enzymes is needed to break down the sucrose in the cake?

    A. Lactase
    C. Peptidase
    B. Maltase
    D. Sucrase

8. What are the four parts of the large intestine in the order from the small intestine to the rectum?

    A. Ascending, transverse, descending, and sigmoid
    B. Descending, transverse, ascending, and sigmoid
    C. Ascending, sigmoid, descending, and transverse
    D. Sigmoid, transverse, descending, and ascending

9. Pregnancy typically is divided into three roughly equal periods of time called _____.

    A. trilogies
    C. semesters
    B. trimesters
    D. menstrual cycles

10. The ovaries are analogous to which component of the male reproductive system?

    A. Foreskin
    C. Sperm
    B. Scrotum
    D. Testis

11. A medical professional needs to perform a macroscopic urinalysis on a patient. Which of the following procedures does she most likely complete?

    A. Compare color of dipstick to a standard chart

    B. Spin down the urine sample using a centrifuge

    C. Analyze for the presence of blood cells in the urine

    D. Prepare a microscope slide using sediments found in the urine

12. After being produced by the kidneys, where does urine flow next?

    A. Ureter   C. Renal vein

    B. Urethra   D. Renal artery

13. Where are blood vessels and nerve fibers found in bone?

    A. Cartilage   C. Spongy bone

    B. Osteocytes   D. Haversian canal

14. Osteoclasts and osteoblasts work together to play a role in bone _____.

    A. mineralization   C. remodeling

    B. ossification   D. resorption

15. Muscles work together in a synchronized fashion through the action of:

    A. opening and closing.

    B. moving up and down.

    C. stretching and pulling.

    D. contracting and extending.

16. Which of the following organs contains cardiac muscle?

    A. Bladder   C. Heart

    B. Brain   D. Skin

17. The hair _____ is not attached to the follicle.

    A. bulb   C. shaft

    B. root   D. strand

18. Squamous cell carcinoma affects cells in the stratum _____.

    A. basale   C. lucidum

    B. granulosum   D. spinosum

19. Epidermal cells are found in the _____ before traveling to the skin's surface.

    A. stratum basale

    B. stratum lucidum

    C. stratum corneum

    D. stratum granulosum

20. Where is genetic information found in a neuron?

    A. Axon   C. Cell body

    B. Dendrite   D. Axon terminal

21. The nervous system works with the endocrine system to

    A. maintain internal homeostasis.

    B. filter wastes and toxins out the body.

    C. protect internal organs from getting damaged.

    D. supply oxygen to the cells and tissues in the body.

105

22. Not all cells in the pancreas secrete insulin because of the hormone somatostatin, which inhibits the release of insulin by all cells. What type of intercellular chemical signal does this illustrate?

    A. Autocrine

    B. Neuromodulator

    C. Paracrine

    D. Pheromone

23. The endocrine system is composed of ductless glands. Why is this efficient?

    A. It enables hormones to be secreted quickly.

    B. It enables hormones to be secreted in minute amounts.

    C. It enables hormones to be secreted directly into the blood.

    D. It enables hormones to be secreted directly onto the target cell.

24. What is usually the first line of defense in the human body when a pathogen invades?

    A. B cell

    B. Macrophage

    C. Mucous covering

    D. T cell

25. Which gland is only active from birth through puberty?

    A. Adenoids   C. Thymus

    B. Appendix   D. Tonsils

SECTION VIII. PHYSICS

You have 50 minutes to complete 25 questions.

1. Which statement best describes the motion of smooth ball thrown into the air on a calm day?

   A. The ball follows a line.

   B. The ball follows a circular path.

   C. The ball follows an erratic path.

   D. The ball follows a parabolic path.

2. Vector $\vec{x}$ has the same length as vector $\vec{y}$ but the exact opposite direction. What is the resultant $\vec{x} + \vec{y}$?

   A. A.$-\vec{x}$

   B. 0

   C. $\frac{1}{2}\vec{x}$

   D. $2\vec{x}$

3. Vector (2, 6) appears on a graph with its tail at (3, 1). What are the coordinates of its head?

   A. (−1, 5)

   B. (1, −5)

   C. (5, 7)

   D. (6, 6)

4. What is the force in the direction (1.0, 2.0) with a magnitude of 3.5 newtons?

   A. (0.45, 0.91) N

   B. (1.6, 3.2) N

   C. (1.9, 3.8) N

   D. (3.5, 7.0) N

5. If a car goes a constant speed of 65 miles per hour over 490 miles, how long is the trip?

   A. 0.13 hours

   B. 7.5 hours

   C. 430 hours

   D. 32,000 hours

6. A softball player throws a ball at a moderately upward angle to the ground. Which term best describes the motion of the ball?

   A. Linear

   B. Nonlinear

   C. Stationary

   D. Rotational

7. Which term best describes the motion of a planet moving at a nonzero speed and a fixed distance from a star?

   A. Linear

   B. Nonlinear

   C. Stationary

   D. Rotational

8. A car at a certain point on a circular racetrack experiences centripetal acceleration to the west. What is the direction of the centripetal acceleration when the car goes halfway around the circle from that point?

   A. East

   B. North

   C. South

   D. West

9. If a stunt airplane pilot is performing a circular loop and at a certain point feels like she is being pushed upward by a force, what is the direction of the centripetal force?

   A. Up

   B. Down

   C. Lateral

   D. Forward

10. An object in uniform circular motion with a radius of 42 meters has an angular frequency of 0.29 hertz. What is its velocity?

    A. 0.0069 m/s

    B. 1.9 m/s

    C. 12 m/s

    D. 140 m/s

11. What differentiates an electromagnetic wave from a mechanical wave?

   A. Only electromagnetic waves can exist in a vacuum.

   B. Only electromagnetic waves can exhibit refraction.

   C. Only electromagnetic waves can travel through a material.

   D. Only electromagnetic waves obey the wave-speed equation $v = \lambda f$.

12. Which two atoms are the same element?

   A. One atom with 4 protons, 4 neutrons, and 3 electrons, and one atom with 3 protons, 4 neutrons, and 3 electrons

   B. One atom with 3 protons, 4 neutrons, and 3 electrons, and one atom with 3 protons, 3 neutrons, and 3 electrons

   C. One atom with 3 protons, 4 neutrons, and 3 electrons, and one atom with 4 protons, 3 neutrons, and 3 electrons

   D. One atom with 4 protons, 4 neutrons, and 3 electrons, and one atom with 3 protons, 3 neutrons, and 4 electrons

13. The maximum speed of light is c. What does this fact imply?

   A. The amplitude of a light wave must be less than 1.

   B. The amplitude of a light wave must be less than the frequency.

   C. The frequency of a light wave must be less than the wavelength.

   D. The refractive index of a material must be greater than or equal to 1.

14. One isotope of a particular element is neutral, and a different isotope of that element is an ion. Which conclusion is correct?

   A. One isotope has more protons than the other.

   B. One isotope has more electrons than the other.

   C. Both isotopes have the same number of neutrons.

   D. Both isotopes have the same number of nucleons.

15. An experimenter has two objects and knows that one of them is positively charged. If that object pushes away the other object when the two are brought into proximity, what can he conclude?

   A. The other object is positively charged.

   B. The other object is negatively charged.

   C. The other object carries no electric charge.

   D. The other object may be either positively or negatively charged.

16. A stationary object can possess which of the following?

   A. Impulse

   B. Momentum

   C. Kinetic energy

   D. Potential energy

17. A carpenter's tool falls off a rooftop and strikes the ground with a certain kinetic energy. If it fell from a roof that was four times higher, how would this new kinetic energy (just before impact) compare to the original roof?

   A. The kinetic energy would be 2 times greater.

   B. The kinetic energy would be 4 times greater.

   C. The kinetic energy would be 8 times greater.

   D. The kinetic energy would be 16 times greater.

18. A bell tower is 52 m tall. The bell weighs 201 N. What type of energy does the bell have?

   A. Chemical
   B. Electrical
   C. Kinetic
   D. Potential

19. If the velocity of an object is decreased by half, by what factor is the kinetic energy reduced?

   A. 2
   B. 4
   C. 6
   D. 8

20. According to Newton's equation for universal gravitation, if the mass of a planet near the sun were tripled,

   A. the force of attraction would be tripled.

   B. the force of attraction would be doubled.

   C. the force of attraction would be quartered.

   D. the force of attraction would be quadrupled.

21. A positive charge and a negative charge are in close proximity. Which statement best describes the field lines around the charges?

   A. No field lines exist between positive and negative charges.

   B. The field lines start at the negative charge and end at the positive charge.

   C. The field lines start at the positive charge and end at the negative charge.

   D. The field lines associated with the positive charge do not connect with the field lines associated with the negative charge.

22. Which of the following will create an electric force around a wire loop?

   A. Constant current inside the loop

   B. Changing electric flux inside the loop

   C. Changing magnetic flux inside the loop

   D. Constant electric and magnetic flux inside the loop

23. The electric force on a 1-coulomb charge is 25 newtons. If that charge is removed, what is the field strength at its former location?

   A. 1 newton per coulomb

   B. 24 newtons per coulomb

   C. 25 newtons per coulomb

   D. 100 newtons per coulomb

24. A proton has an electron on either side of it such that all three particles lie on a line and each electron is 1 millimeter from the proton. What is the direction of the net electric force on the proton?

   A. No net force acts on the proton.

   B. The force is toward one of the electrons.

   C. Electrons and protons exert no electric force on each other.

   D. The force is perpendicular to the line on which the three particles lie.

25. What is the electric field 3.0×10^2 meters from a 5.0×10^{-3}-coulomb charge? (Assume the electric constant is 9×10^9 when using units of newtons, coulombs, and meters.)

   A. 2.5 newtons per coulomb

   B. 5.0×10^2 newtons per coulomb

   C. 1.5×10^5 newtons per coulomb

   D. 2.3×10^5 newtons per coulomb

HESI Practice Exam 2
Answer Key with Explanatory Answers

Section I. Mathematics

1. **C.** The correct solution is adding two quantities with different units. To add quantities, they must have the same unit. For instance, adding a quantity of meters to a quantity of grams is impossible. **Skill: Basic Addition and Subtraction.**

2. **C.** The correct solution is –561. Start at 0 on the number line and go 561 steps to the left, ending at –561. Or note that 0 – 561 = –(561 – 0) = –561. **Skill: Basic Addition and Subtraction.**

3. **D.** The correct solution is 20 > –21. When in doubt, draw a number line and place the numbers on it, recalling that greater numbers are farther right than lesser numbers. Here, note that because a positive number is always greater than a negative number, 20 > –21. **Skill: Basic Addition and Subtraction.**

4. **A.** The correct solution is –1. This subtraction is easy to see on a number line or by inspection because the numbers are close. Remember that when subtracting a larger number from a smaller one, the difference is negative. **Skill: Basic Addition and Subtraction.**

5. **D.** The correct solution is none of the above. The complete number line comprises all possible numbers, including fraction/decimal numbers. This is an infinite number of numbers. **Skill: Basic Addition and Subtraction.**

6. **C.** Follow the order of operations (the PEMDAS mnemonic). Begin with the innermost parentheses and work outward, multiplying and dividing from left to right before adding and subtracting from left to right.

$(3 \times (4 + 9) \div 13 - 2) + 1$
$(3 \times 13 \div 13 - 2) + 1$
$(39 \div 13 - 2) + 1$
$(3 - 2) + 1$
$1 + 1$
2

Skill: Basic Multiplication and Division.

7. **D.** Use the multiplication algorithm. It involves adding 40 and 80 to get the product of 120. **Skill: Basic Multiplication and Division.**

8. **C.** When dividing signed numbers, remember that if the dividend and divisor have the same sign, the quotient is positive. Other than the sign, the process is the same as dividing whole numbers. **Skill: Basic Multiplication and Division.**

9. A. The order of operations (recall the mnemonic PEMDAS) requires multiplication and division before addition and subtraction. **Skill: Basic Multiplication and Division.**

10. B. Use division, ignoring the remainder (which is how much Linda has left after paying $5 per widget). In this case, $321 \div 5 = 64R1$. She can buy 64 widgets. **Skill: Basic Multiplication and Division.**

11. D. The correct solution is 1.8057 because 1.8057 contains the largest value in the tenths place. **Skill: Decimals and Fractions.**

12. A. The correct solution is $\frac{3}{8}$ because $\frac{0.375}{1} = \frac{375}{1000} = \frac{3}{8}$. **Skill: Decimals and Fractions.**

13. D. The correct solution is $2\frac{1}{2}$ because $2\frac{0.5}{1} = 2\frac{5}{10} = 2\frac{1}{2}$. **Skill: Decimals and Fractions.**

14. C. The correct answer is $\frac{1}{8}$ because 12.5% as a fraction is $\frac{12.5}{100} = \frac{125}{1000} = \frac{1}{8}$. **Skill: Decimals and Fractions.**

15. A. The correct answer is 1.455 because 145.5% as a decimal is $145.5 \div 100 = 1.455$. **Skill: Decimals and Fractions.**

16. B. The correct solution is −10 because 10 is added to both sides of the equation. **Skill: Equations with One Variable.**

17. C. The correct solution is $\frac{y-b}{m} = x$.

$$y-b = mx$$ 　　　　　Subtract b from both sides of the equation.

$$\frac{y-b}{m} = x$$

Divide both sides of the equation by m.

Skill: Equations with One Variable.

18. A. The correct solution is $x < \frac{2}{5}$.

$2(4x + 3) < 3x + 8$	Multiply all terms by the least common denominator of 4 to eliminate the fractions.
$8x + 6 < 3x + 8$	Apply the distributive property.
$5x + 6 < 8$	Subtract $3x$ from both sides of the inequality.
$5x < 2$	Subtract 6 from both sides of the inequality.
$x < \frac{2}{5}$	Divide both sides of the inequality by 5.

Skill: Equations with One Variable.

19. C. The correct solution is $\frac{2}{3}$.

$3x + 2 + 9 = 6x + 9$	Multiply all terms by the least common denominator of 3 to eliminate the fractions.
$3x + 11 = 6x + 9$	Combine like terms on the left side of the equation.
$-3x + 11 = 9$	Subtract $6x$ from both sides of the equation.
$-3x = -2$	Subtract 11 from both sides of the equation.
$x = \frac{2}{3}$	Divide both sides of the equation by -3.

Skill: Equations with One Variable.

20. A. The correct solutions are (1, -2) and (-1, 2).

$x^2 + (-2x)^2 = 5$	Substitute $-2x$ in for y in the second equation.
$x^2 + 4x^2 = 5$	Apply the exponent.
$5x^2 = 5$	Combine like terms on the left side of the equation.
$x^2 = 1$	Divide both sides of the equation by 5.
$x = \pm 1$	Apply the square root to both sides of the equation.
$y = -2(1) = -2$	Substitute 1 in the first equation and multiply.
$y = -2(-1) = 2$	Substitute -1 in the first equation and multiply.

Skill: Equations with Two Variables.

21. D. The correct solutions are (1, 4) and (-1, -4).

$x^2 + (4x)^2 = 17$	Substitute $4x$ in for y in the second equation.
$x^2 + 16x^2 = 17$	Apply the exponent.
$17x^2 = 17$	Combine like terms on the left side of the equation.
$x^2 = 1$	Divide both sides of the equation by 17.
$x = \pm 1$	Apply the square root to both sides of the equation.
$y = 4(1) = 4$	Substitute 1 in the first equation and multiply.
$y = 4(-1) = -4$	Substitute -1 in the first equation and multiply.

Skill: Equations with Two Variables.

22. B. The correct solutions are (-1.4, 4.2) and (1.4, -4.2).

$x^2 + (-3x)^2 = 20$	Substitute $-3x$ in for y in the second equation.
$x^2 + 9x^2 = 20$	Apply the exponent.
$10x^2 = 20$	Combine like terms on the left side of the equation.
$x^2 = 2$	Divide both sides of the equation by 10.
$x = \pm 1.4$	Apply the square root to both sides of the equation.
$y = -3(1.4) = -4.2$	Substitute 1.4 in the first equation and multiply.
$y = -3(-1.4) = 4.2$	Substitute -1.4 in the first equation and multiply.

Skill: Equations with Two Variables.

23. A. The correct solution is (2, 4).

$25x + 15y = 110$	Multiply all terms in the first equation by 5.
$6x{-}15y = -48$	Multiply all terms in the second equation by 3.
$31x = 62$	Add the equations.
$x = 2$	Divide both sides of the equation by 31.
$5(2) + 3y = 22$	Substitute 2 in the first equation for x.
$10 + 3y = 22$	Simplify using order of operations.
$3y = 12$	Subtract 10 from both sides of the equation.
$y = 4$	Divide both sides of the equation by 3.

Skill: Equations with Two Variables.

24. A. The correct answer is $\frac{20}{43}$ because $\frac{5}{3} \div \frac{43}{12} = \frac{5}{3} \times \frac{12}{43} = \frac{60}{129} = \frac{20}{43}$. **Skill: Multiplication and Division of Fractions.**

25. D. The correct solution is $9\frac{3}{8}$ because $\frac{5}{2} \times \frac{15}{4} = \frac{75}{8} = 9\frac{3}{8}$. **Skill: Multiplication and Division of Fractions.**

26. D. The correct answer is $8\frac{2}{3}$ because $\frac{13}{7} \div \frac{3}{14} = \frac{13}{7} \times \frac{14}{3} = \frac{182}{21} = 8\frac{14}{21} = 8\frac{2}{3}$. **Skill: Multiplication and Division of Fractions.**

27. D. The correct solution is $8\frac{2}{3}$ because $\frac{13}{4} \times \frac{8}{3} = \frac{104}{12} = 8\frac{8}{12} = 8\frac{2}{3}$. **Skill: Multiplication and Division of Fractions.**

28. D. The correct solution is $y^3 - 4y^2 + 9y + 3$.

$$(3y^3 - 4y^2 + 6y + 3) - (2y^3 - 3y) = (3y^3 - 4y^2 + 6y + 3) + (-2y^3 + 3y)$$
$$= (3y^3 - 2y^3) - 4y^2 + (6y + 3y) + 3 = y^3 - 4y^2 + 9y + 3$$

Skill: Polynomials.

29. D. The correct solution is $6x^2y^2-7xy + 2$.

$(2xy-1)(3xy-2) = (2xy)(3xy-2)-1(3xy-2) = 6x^2y^2-4xy-3xy + 2 = 6x^2y^2-7xy + 2$

Skill: Polynomials.

30. B. The correct solution is $x-xy-2y$.

$(8x + 2xy-4y) + (-7x-3xy + 2y) = (8x-7x) + (2xy-3xy) + (-4y + 2y) = x-xy-2y$

Skill: Polynomials.

31. D. The correct solution is $-5y^3 + 5y^2 + 4y-3$.

$(3y^2 + 4y)-(5y^3-2y^2 + 3) = (3y^2 + 4y) + (-5y^3 + 2y^2-3)$
$= -5y^3 + (3y^2 + 2y^2) + 4y-3 = -5y^3 + 5y^2 + 4y-3$

Skill: Polynomials.

32. B. The correct solution is $5x^3-2x^2-4x-1$.

$(5x^3 + 3x^2-4x + 2) + (-5x^2-3) = 5x^3 + (3x^2-5x^2)-4x + (2-3)$
$= 5x^3-2x^2-4x-1$

Skill: Polynomials.

33. C. The correct solution is $\frac{x^{25}}{y^{25}}$ because

$\left(\frac{x^3y^{-2}}{x^{-2}y^3}\right)^5 = \left(x^{3-(-2)}y^{-2-3}\right)^5 = (x^5y^{-5})^5 = x^{5\times5}y^{-5\times5} = x^{25}y^{-25} = \frac{x^{25}}{y^{25}}$.

Skill: Powers, Exponents, Roots, and Radicals.

34. C. The correct solution is $\frac{x^2}{z^4}$ because

$\left(\frac{xy^0}{z^2}\right)^2 = \frac{x^{1\times2}y^{0\times2}}{z^{2\times2}} = \frac{x^2y^0}{z^4} = \frac{x^2}{z^4}$.

Skill: Powers, Exponents, Roots, and Radicals.

35. A. The correct solution is $\frac{1}{16}$ because

$\left((2^{-2})^{-1}\right)^{-2} = 2^{-2\times(-1)\times(-2)} = 2^{-4} = \frac{1}{2^4} = \frac{1}{16}$.

Skill: Powers, Exponents, Roots, and Radicals.

36. B. The correct solution is -2 because the cube root of -8 is -2. **Skill: Powers, Exponents, Roots, and Radicals.**

37. C. The fraction $\frac{22}{54}$ is 41%, meaning 22 is 41% of 54. **Skill: Ratios, Proportions, and Percentages.**

38. B. The correct answer is B. Set up the proportion of dogs to cats (or vice versa):

$$\frac{2}{3} = \frac{?}{1,425}$$

Since $1,425 \div 3 = 475$, the number of dogs is the product of 2 and 475, or 950. **Skill: Ratios, Proportions, and Percentages.**

39. C. The company employs 273 men. If 35% of the company's employees are women, 65% are men. Set up a proportion using 65%, which is equal to $\frac{65}{100}$ or $\frac{13}{20}$:

$$\frac{13}{20} = \frac{?}{420}$$

The unknown number is the product of 13 and $420 \div 20 = 21$, which is 273. **Skill: Ratios, Proportions, and Percentages.**

40. D. The truck has a 67% change in speed. The truck's change in speed is the difference between its final and initial speed: in this case, 100 mph − 60 mph = 40 mph. To find the percent change, divide 40 mph by the initial speed (60 mph) and then multiply by 100%.

$$\frac{40 \; mph}{60 \; mph} \times 100\% = 0.67 \times 100\% = 67\%$$

Skill: Ratios, Proportions, and Percentages.

41. A. The company's revenue is decreasing −$60 million in a year. Begin by calculating the revenue decrease, which is the difference between $118 million and $123 million, or −$5 million. That decrease is for one month. Next, set up a proportion to find the equivalent rate of change for a year, noting that a year is 12 months:

$$\frac{-\$5 \; million}{1 \; month} = \frac{?}{12 \; months}$$

Because the denominator on the right is 12 times the denominator on the left, find the unknown rate of change by multiplying −$5 million by 12 to get −$60 million. Because the question asked for a rate of increase but the revenue is decreasing, the negative sign is critical. **Skill: Ratios, Proportions, and Percentages.**

42. D. The correct solution is $38\frac{8}{15}$ because

$$15\frac{3}{5} + 3\frac{2}{3} = 15\frac{9}{15} + 3\frac{10}{15} = 18\frac{19}{15}(2) = \frac{289}{15} \times \frac{2}{1} = \frac{578}{15} = 38\frac{8}{15} \text{ feet.}$$

Skill: Solving Real World Mathematical Problems.

43. B. The correct solution is 20.48 because 39.45–18.97 = 20.48 feet. **Skill: Solving Real World Mathematical Problems.**

44. B. The correct solution is $4\frac{5}{12}$ because $5\frac{2}{3}-1\frac{1}{4} = 5\frac{8}{12}-1\frac{3}{12} = 4\frac{5}{12}$ feet. **Skill: Solving Real World Mathematical Problems.**

45. C. The correct solution is $7\frac{7}{12}$ because $3\frac{1}{3} + 2\frac{1}{2} + 1\frac{3}{4} = 3\frac{4}{12} + 2\frac{6}{12} + 1\frac{9}{12} = 6\frac{19}{12} = 7\frac{7}{12}$ yards of fabric. **Skill: Solving Real World Mathematical Problems.**

46. D. The correct solution is 48.6 because 5.4(3)(3) = 48.6 gallons. **Skill: Solving Real World Mathematical Problems.**

47. B. The correct solution is 500,000 milliliters. $0.5\ kL \times \frac{1,000\ L}{1\ kL} \times \frac{1,000\ mL}{1\ L} = 500,000\ mL$. **Skill: Standards of Measure.**

48. B. The correct solution is 0.795 quarts. $750\ mL \times \frac{1\ L}{1,000\ mL} \times \frac{1.06\ qt}{1\ L} = \frac{795}{1000} = 0.795\ qt$. **Skill: Standards of Measure.**

49. A. The correct solution is 4.25 liters. $9\ pt \times \frac{1\ qt}{2\ pt} \times \frac{1\ L}{1.06\ qt} = \frac{9}{2.12} = 4.25\ L$. **Skill: Standards of Measure.**

50. B. The correct solution is 28.98 kilometers. $18\ mi \times \frac{1.61\ km}{1\ mi} = 28.98\ km$. **Skill: Standards of Measure.**

Section II. Reading Comprehension

1. B. All of the above sentences relate to author income, and particularly to differences in income for male and female authors. **Skill: Main Ideas, Topic Sentences, and Supporting Details.**

2. B. The sentences above discuss pay differences between male and female authors but not differences in the quality or appeal of their work, so the best topic sentence would relate to gender stereotyping and author pay. **Skill: Main Ideas, Topic Sentences, and Supporting Details.**

3. D. The collection of sentences above all relate to gender differences in author income, so the best fit for the topic is a statement about people's likelihood of purchasing books by men and women. **Skill: Main Ideas, Topic Sentences, and Supporting Details.**

4. B. This passage argues that teens and young adults spend too much time on social media. **Skill: Facts Opinions and Evaluating an Argument.**

5. B. Factual information is verifiable and not based on personal beliefs or feelings. The statistic about the number of teens who go online daily is a fact. **Skill: Facts Opinions and Evaluating an Argument.**

6. A. This statement takes a complex issue and presents it as if only two possible options are in play. This is an either/or fallacy. **Skill: Facts Opinions and Evaluating an Argument.**

7. B. This sentence makes an overgeneralization by claiming that online interactions are never as good as conversations with human beings. It is possible to imagine many exceptions to this statement. **Skill: Facts Opinions and Evaluating an Argument.**

8. C. The sentence in question is an example of circular reasoning. That is, it restates the argument in different words instead of providing evidence to back it up. **Skill: Facts Opinions and Evaluating an Argument.**

9. A. The phrase "too much" in this sentence reflects a judgment that is subject to interpretation. This indicates that the sentence reflects a belief rather than a fact. **Skill: Facts Opinions and Evaluating an Argument.**

10. A. Passage 1 is intended to inform readers about electroconvulsive therapy. **Skill: Understanding the Author's Purpose, Point of View, and Rhetorical Strategies.**

11. C. The second paragraph of passage 1 makes opinion statements about what doctors should do. This is a sign of persuasive writing. **Skill: Understanding the Author's Purpose, Point of View, and Rhetorical Strategies.**

12. D. Passage 2 tells a story, which is meant to entertain. **Skill: Understanding the Author's Purpose, Point of View, and Rhetorical Strategies.**

13. D. Passage 1 says that electroconvulsive therapy is "a genuine option for patients whose symptoms do not improve with medication." This suggests that medication should be tried first. **Skill: Understanding the Author's Purpose, Point of View, and Rhetorical Strategies.**

14. C. The detail about electroconvulsive therapy as "a genuine option for patients whose symptoms do not improve with medication" suggests that patients should try an option like medication first, before contemplating electroconvulsive therapy. **Skill: Understanding the Author's Purpose, Point of View, and Rhetorical Strategies.**

15. A. The author of Passage 2 is aware that many people have negative preconceived ideas about electroconvulsive therapy. This is true of the author of Passage 2, who does not inform herself about the facts of the situation. **Skill: Understanding the Author's Purpose, Point of View, and Rhetorical Strategies.**

16. D. The author of Passage 1 specifically recommends extra care in communication about electroconvulsive therapy. The doctor in Passage 2 does not seem to make any extra effort to differentiate between myth and reality. **Skill: Understanding the Author's Purpose, Point of View, and Rhetorical Strategies.**

17. A. The author of Passage 2 describes doctors blocking her "direct path to the door," which suggests that she feels trapped in the room. This suggests a negative, fearful outlook which is further reinforced by the comment about Big Doctor being "sadistic." **Skill: Understanding the Author's Purpose, Point of View, and Rhetorical Strategies.**

18. B. The author of Passage 1 uses primarily facts and logic, although she could strengthen her points by clearly identifying sources or establishing her credentials. **Skill: Understanding the Author's Purpose, Point of View, and Rhetorical Strategies.**

19. C. The topic of this paragraph is related to obesity, but it is more narrowly focused on the fad diets people use as they try to control their weight. **Skill: Main Ideas, Topic Sentences, and Supporting Details.**

20. A. The first sentence of this paragraph leads the reader toward the main idea, which is expressed next in a topic sentence about the harmfulness of fad diets. **Skill: Main Ideas, Topic Sentences, and Supporting Details.**

21. C. A description of a failed experience with fad diets would function as a supporting detail in this paragraph about the negative consequences of fad diets. **Skill: Main Ideas, Topic Sentences, and Supporting Details.**

22. B. Although this description of the paragraph would be valid in an opinion response, it is not merely a statement of the main idea because it adds the reader's judgment about the paragraph. **Skill: Main Ideas, Topic Sentences, and Supporting Details.**

23. A. Although a statistic about early childhood obesity might belong in a passage focusing on obesity rates, it would be off-topic information in this paragraph on the harm of fad dieting. **Skill: Main Ideas, Topic Sentences, and Supporting Details.**

24. A. This author is not very trustworthy, but he does not make any attempt to conceal the fact that he is sharing his personal opinions rather than facts. The fact that he begins with the sentence "You know what I hate?" is a clear cue that this is argumentative writing. **Skill: Understanding Primary Sources Making Inferences and Drawing Conclusions.**

25. C. The sentence about freelancers not making as much money is one of the few logical points this blog post makes, but the writer does not share his sources. This makes it difficult for the reader to verify the information. **Skill: Understanding Primary Sources Making Inferences and Drawing Conclusions.**

26. B. The passage raises the opposing argument that freelancing provides greater freedom for workers, but the writer does not respond to this argument. Instead, he makes a manipulatively emotional argument. **Skill: Understanding Primary Sources Making Inferences and Drawing Conclusions.**

27. C. A government website tracking statistics might be a good source, but it would provide facts rather than opinions. An opinion article by an expert in the field would more likely offer what the student is looking for. **Skill: Understanding Primary Sources Making Inferences and Drawing Conclusions.**

28. B. A summary must restate the ideas of the original text, not comment on them with judgments or speculation, and without adhering too closely to the wording of the original. This paragraph explains how shipping and refrigeration technology helped bananas become a major export crop. **Skill: Summarizing Text and Using Text Features.**

29. B. These sentences, like all effective summaries, restate the ideas of the original text in different words. Although a summary can sometimes state an implicit idea from the original text, this one does not need to do so. **Skill: Summarizing Text and Using Text Features.**

30. C. The structure and word choice of this sentence are so close to the original that it qualifies as plagiarism. **Skill: Summarizing Text and Using Text Features.**

31. B. This sentence comments on the original text rather than summarizing it. Some types of writing allow this, but it is not a summary. **Skill: Summarizing Text and Using Text Features.**

32. D. It would be inaccurate to say that nobody would eat bananas if modern shipping and refrigeration technology had never been invented. This is not in the original text, and logically speaking, bananas would still be eaten in the tropics regardless of changes in technology. **Skill: Summarizing Text and Using Text Features.**

33. B. The tone of this letter is hostile and arrogant as the author openly assumes her wealth and influence will secure a good chemistry grade for her daughter. **Skill: Tone and Mood, Transition Words.**

34. C. The author of the letter uses mostly polite language to make her arrogant request, but her language becomes openly hostile when she calls grading practices "petty" and accuses Dr. Rodriguez of being "incompetent." **Skill: Tone and Mood, Transition Words.**

35. A. A teacher receiving a note like this would likely feel furious. **Skill: Tone and Mood, Transition Words.**

36. C. The phrase "in fact" adds emphasis to the writer's implicit point that she intends to make sure her daughter unfairly receives a high chemistry grade. **Skill: Tone and Mood, Transition Words.**

37. C. This passage ironically is a humorous description of a toddler's emotions, written by an adult who has enough experience to know that a toddler's huge emotions will pass. **Skill: Tone and Mood, Transition Words.**

38. B. Authors use irony when their words do not literally mean what they say. The joy does not really go out of the world when a toddler loses her binky—but it may seem that way to the child. **Skill: Tone and Mood, Transition Words.**

39. B. This passage establishes irony in the opening sentence by applying the superlative phrase "the most amazing thing ever" to an ordinary occurrence. **Skill: Tone and Mood, Transition Words.**

40. A. Effective readers would likely know that this toddler's fear is nothing to worry about. Amusement would be a more likely reaction. **Skill: Tone and Mood, Transition Words.**

41. B. The word "below" in paragraph one provides information about where the train is situated in relation to the character. It does not transition between ideas. **Skill: Tone and Mood, Transition Words.**

42. A. "Later" and "afterward" are both time/sequence transitions that show when events happen in relation to one another. **Skill: Tone and Mood, Transition Words.**

43. C. This passage shares the author's opinions about television and movie rating systems. This makes it a persuasive piece. **Skill: Understanding the Author's Purpose, Point of View, and Rhetorical Strategies.**

44. D. The author of the passage says that only she knows her kids well enough to be able to decide what they can watch. She would likely agree that other parents are the best people to make similar choices for their own kids. **Skill: Understanding the Author's Purpose, Point of View, and Rhetorical Strategies.**

45. C. The author of this passage suggests that parents should decide for themselves whether or not kids should watch certain shows or movies. She would likely agree with an effort to provide parents more information for making these choices. **Skill: Understanding the Author's Purpose, Point of View, and Rhetorical Strategies.**

46. D. The author includes her credentials as a parent to establish that she is a trustworthy authority on this subject. **Skill: Understanding the Author's Purpose, Point of View, and Rhetorical Strategies.**

47. C. The author uses the phrase "based on numbers" in a negative way, she is implying that some decisions need to be based on more nuanced positions. **Skill: Understanding the Author's Purpose, Point of View, and Rhetorical Strategies.**

Section III. Vocabulary & General Knowledge

1. B. The suffix that means "capable of" is *tion*. **Skill: Root Words, Prefixes, and Suffixes.**

2. B. The suffix that means "happened in the past" is *ed*. **Skill: Root Words, Prefixes, and Suffixes.**

3. D. The suffix that means "the study of" is *logy*. **Skill: Root Words, Prefixes, and Suffixes.**

4. A. The root that means "to throw" is *ject*. **Skill: Root Words, Prefixes, and Suffixes.**

5. D. The root that means "to build" is *struct*. **Skill: Root Words, Prefixes, and Suffixes.**

6. C. The prefix that means "water" is *hydro*. **Skill: Root Words, Prefixes, and Suffixes.**

7. C. The root *multi* means "many," so multifaceted means having many sides. **Skill: Root Words, Prefixes, and Suffixes.**

8. B. The root *sect* means "cut," so dissect means to separate, or cut, into pieces. **Skill: Root Words, Prefixes, and Suffixes.**

9. A. The suffix *ous* means "full of or possessing " so a parsimonious person is one who is full of stinginess. **Skill: Root Words, Prefixes, and Suffixes.**

10. C. The prefix that means "incorrect" is *mis*. **Skill: Root Words, Prefixes, and Suffixes.**

11. D. The root *pug* means "war," or "fight," so pugnacious means combative. **Skill: Root Words, Prefixes, and Suffixes.**

12. D. The prefix *sub* means "below," so a subservient person would be obedient to someone else. **Skill: Root Words, Prefixes, and Suffixes.**

13. D. The root *rupt* means "break," so rupture means to burst. **Skill: Root Words, Prefixes, and Suffixes.**

14. C. The prefix that means "between" is *inter*. **Skill: Root Words, Prefixes, and Suffixes.**

15. B. The prefix *pre* means "before," so a premonition means something is known before it happens. **Skill: Root Words, Prefixes, and Suffixes.**

16. C. The prefix that means "self" is *auto*. **Skill: Root Words, Prefixes, and Suffixes.**

17. D. The root *cred* means "believe," the prefix *in* means "not," and the suffix *ous* means "full of or possessing," so, incredulous means disbelieving. **Skill: Root Words, Prefixes, and Suffixes.**

18. A. The prefix *re* means "again," so reinstate would be to get the "state" of the person's position again or to restore that person's position. **Skill: Root Words, Prefixes, and Suffixes.**

19. D. The prefix *trans* means "across," and the root word *luc* means "light," so translucent means letting some light to pass through or across. **Skill: Root Words, Prefixes, and Suffixes.**

20. C. The prefix *mis* means "wrong," so a miscreant would be someone who does something wrong. Villainous is the best answer. **Skill: Root Words, Prefixes, and Suffixes.**

21. B. The root word *veri* means "true," so veritable means genuine. **Skill: Root Words, Prefixes, and Suffixes.**

22. C. The prefix that means "with" is *con*. **Skill: Root Words, Prefixes, and Suffixes.**

23. C. The root that means "color" is *chrom*. **Skill: Root Words, Prefixes, and Suffixes.**

24. C. The meaning of <u>hatch</u> in this context is "to create or produce an idea in a secret way." The word "plan" helps you figure out which meaning of <u>hatch</u> is being used. **Skill: Context Clues and Multiple Meaning Words.**

25. C. The meaning of <u>operation</u> in this context is "a small business." The phrase "worked" helps you figure out which meaning of <u>operation</u> is being used. **Skill: Context Clues and Multiple Meaning Words.**

26. D. The meaning of <u>bass</u> in the context of this sentence is "a guitar with four strings that makes low sounds." **Skill: Context Clues and Multiple Meaning Words.**

27. B. The meaning of <u>bolt</u> in the context of this sentence is "a quick movement in a particular direction. **Skill: Context Clues and Multiple Meaning Words.**

28. C. The meaning of <u>unkempt</u> in this context is "messy or untidy." The phrase "knickknacks strewn" helps you figure out the meaning of <u>unkempt</u>. **Skill: Context Clues and Multiple Meaning Words.**

29. A. The meaning of <u>base</u> in the context of this sentence is "the bottom or lowest part of something." **Skill: Context Clues and Multiple Meaning Words.**

30. B. The meaning of <u>facetious</u> in this context is "treating serious issues with inappropriate humor." The word "smirked" helps you figure out the meaning of <u>facetious</u>. **Skill: Context Clues and Multiple Meaning Words.**

31. A. The meaning of <u>harbor</u> in the context of this sentence is "to hide someone." **Skill: Context Clues and Multiple Meaning Words.**

32. C. The meaning of <u>emulate</u> in this context is "to try to be like someone you admire." The word "imitate" helps you figure out the meaning of <u>emulate</u>. **Skill: Context Clues and Multiple Meaning Words.**

33. D. The meaning of <u>reconnaissance</u> in this context is "military activity in which groups are sent out to get information about an enemy." The word "enemy" helps you figure out the meaning of <u>reconnaissance</u>. **Skill: Context Clues and Multiple Meaning Words.**

34. B. The meaning of <u>draft</u> in the context of this sentence is "a version of a document such as a written paper." **Skill: Context Clues and Multiple Meaning Words.**

35. A. The meaning of <u>crop</u> in the context of this sentence is "to cut off a part of." **Skill: Context Clues and Multiple Meaning Words.**

36. D. The meaning of <u>pungent</u> in this context is "having a strong smell." The word "tear" helps you figure out the meaning of <u>pungent</u>. **Skill: Context Clues and Multiple Meaning Words.**

37. B. The meaning of <u>program</u> in this context is "something that is broadcast on television or radio." The phrase "watched" helps you figure out which meaning of <u>program</u> is being used. **Skill: Context Clues and Multiple Meaning Words.**

38. C. Adding the prefix "para" would make the word "parathyroid," or the area beside or next to the thyroid. **Skill: Domain-Specific Words: Medical Industry.**

39. A. "Myopathy" is a disease of the muscle or muscle tissue. **Skill: Domain-Specific Words: Medical Industry.**

40. B. "Neurology" is the study of the nervous system. **Skill: Domain-Specific Words: Medical Industry.**

41. C. "Gastr" pertains to the stomach, so the patient was experiencing stomach pain. **Skill: Domain-Specific Words: Medical Industry.**

42. A. "Cytology" is the study of the structure and function of cells. **Skill: Domain-Specific Words: Medical Industry.**

43. B. A "nephrectomy" is a procedure conducted to remove a kidney. **Skill: Domain-Specific Words: Medical Industry.**

44. A. "Ocular" pertains to the eye, so the patient is taking eye medicine. **Skill: Domain-Specific Words: Medical Industry.**

45. C. "Hemotoxic" means blood poisoning. **Skill: Domain-Specific Words: Medical Industry.**

46. B. The word "epidermis" means "the outer layer of skin." **Skill: Domain-Specific Words: Medical Industry.**

47. A. Pneum or pneumon refers to the "lung," so the surgeon will excise the patient's lung. **Skill: Domain-Specific Words: Medical Industry.**

48. B. An "endoscopy" is a viewing of the inside of a patient's body to see his/her internal parts. **Skill: Domain-Specific Words: Medical Industry.**

49. A. "Hepa" refers to the "liver," so the patient was suffering from inflammation of the liver. **Skill: Domain-Specific Words: Medical Industry.**

50. A. An "osteocytes" are bone cells. **Skill: Domain-Specific Words: Medical Industry.**

Section IV. Grammar

1. C. With a word ending in -sh, add -es. **Skill: Spelling.**

2. C. With a word ending in -y, you drop the -y and add -ies. **Skill: Spelling.**

3. D. *Bear* is the correctly spelled form of the animal. **Skill: Spelling.**

4. D. *Read* is the action of reading and is correctly spelled. **Skill: Spelling.**

5. D. Harry Potter and the Prisoner of Azkaban. Short prepositions, conjunctions, and articles are not capitalized in publication titles. **Skill: Capitalization.**

6. B. *Northern Ireland.* Directional words like northern are capitalized when it is a part of the official name. **Skill: Capitalization.**

7. A. *southern California.* Words such as southern are not capitalized unless they are a part of the official name. States are always capitalized. **Skill: Capitalization.**

8. C. *Philadelphia Eagles, New England Patriots.* Cities, regions, and sports teams are meant to be capitalized. **Skill: Capitalization.**

9. A. *Highestranking needs a hyphen.* Hyphens are used for compound words that describe a person or object. **Skill: Punctuation.**

10. C. *State of the art should be hyphenated.* It is a compound word before a noun and needs to be hyphenated. **Skill: Punctuation.**

11. **A.** *Elizabeths needs an apostrophe.* Apostrophes indicate possession and the grandsons belong to her. **Skill: Punctuation.**

12. **D.** *There should be commas before and after unfortunately.* Commas are used to set off thoughts and emotions. **Skill: Punctuation.**

13. **A.** *Knives* is the plural form of knife. *Salmon* is a non-count noun, so it does not have a plural form. **Skill: Nouns.**

14. **B.** *Susan* is a noun; the other answers have pronouns as their subjects. **Skill: Nouns.**

15. **C.** *a lot of homework. Homework* is a non-count noun and cannot be made plural by adding -s. **Skill: Nouns.**

16. **C.** *Ivana, Helen*, and *Tony* are nouns. Sentence a has one noun (ice), b has two nouns (weddings, occasions), and d has two nouns (Hitoshi, San Francisco). **Skill: Nouns.**

17. **D.** *Who* is a relative pronoun that refers to the subject *Greta Garbo*. **Skill: Pronouns.**

18. **B.** *Mine* refers to *exams*. **Skill: Pronouns.**

19. **B.** *Them* refers to *fish*. **Skill: Pronouns.**

20. **D.** These adjectives describe *Henry*. **Skill:** Adjectives and Adverbs.

21. **B.** *So* is an adverb that describes the adverb *hard*. (*Hard* describes the verb *hit*.) **Skill:** Adjectives and Adverbs.

22. **C.** *Difficult* is an adjective that describes the noun *homework*. **Skill:** Adjectives and Adverbs.

23. **D.** *Merrily* is an adverb that describes the verb *roll*. **Skill:** Adjectives and Adverbs.

24. **D.** *In, of,* and *on* are prepositions in the other titles. **Skill: Conjunctions and Prepositions.**

25. **C.** *But* and *yet* have the same meaning here. **Skill: Conjunctions and Prepositions.**

26. **C.** *And* is a conjunction. **Skill: Conjunctions and Prepositions.**

27. **A.** *Either/or* is a correlative conjunction pair that can connect *at your office* and *at the station*. **Skill: Conjunctions and Prepositions.**

28. **B.** *Offered* and *advised* are simple past tense verb forms. **Skill: Verbs and Verb Tenses.**

29. **C.** *Was unfolding* (past progressive) is the correct verb tense to use in this sentence. **Skill: Verbs and Verb Tenses.**

30. **B.** This sentence is in simple present tense, and it describes something that happens regularly. **Skill: Verbs and Verb Tenses.**

31. **B.** This sentence has a predicate within a predicate. The "inside" predicate is *who I have visited for years*, and the "outside" predicate is *my dentist has suddenly disappeared*. **Skill: Subject and Verb Agreement.**

32. C. *Meteorologist announces* and *hurricane is* have the correct subject-verb agreement. **Skill: Subject and Verb Agreement.**

33. B. The subject *news* is third person singular, so it takes the verb *was*. **Skill: Subject and Verb Agreement.**

34. C. *Box* is a third person singular subject, so it takes the verb form *needs*. *Of toys* is a prepositional phrase; it is not the subject. **Skill: Subject and Verb Agreement.**

35. C. This sentence correctly fixes the fragment. **Skill: Types of Sentences.**

36. C. This is a compound sentence joining two independent clauses with a comma and the conjunction *and*. **Skill: Types of Sentences.**

37. C. This is a compound sentence joining two independent clauses with a comma and the conjunction *so*. **Skill: Types of Sentences.**

38. B. This is a complex sentence because it starts with a subordinating conjunction, *after*, has a dependent clause followed by a comma, and then has an independent clause. **Skill: Types of Sentences.**

39. D. Unless. The word "unless" signifies the beginning of a dependent clause and is the only conjunction that makes sense in the sentence. **Skill: Types of Clauses.**

40. C. Which. The word "which" signifies the beginning of a dependent clause and is the only conjunction that makes sense in the sentence. **Skill: Types of Clauses.**

41. A. If. The word "if" signifies the beginning of a dependent clause and is the only conjunction that makes sense in the sentence. **Skill: Types of Clauses.**

42. D. Although. The word "although" signifies the beginning of a dependent clause and is the only conjunction that makes sense in the sentence. **Skill: Types of Clauses.**

43. D. *Which was ugly* most likely refers to *hat*, so it should be placed after that word, not after *head*. **Skill: Modifiers, misplaced modifiers, dangling modifiers.**

44. A. Of these choices, *after eating* can only reference *we*. **Skill: Modifiers, misplaced modifiers, dangling modifiers.**

45. B. *Spinning their web* should modify *spiders*, but here it is misplaced to modify *I*. **Skill: Modifiers, misplaced modifiers, dangling modifiers.**

46. C. *That I wrote on the Korean War* should modify *report*, so it should be placed after that word. **Skill: Modifiers, misplaced modifiers, dangling modifiers.**

47. C. *A movie* is the direct object of the verb *watched*. **Skill: Direct Objects and Indirect Objects.**

48. D. There is no indirect object. **Skill: Direct Objects and Indirect Objects.**

49. C. *Portrait* is the direct object of the verb *painted*. **Skill: Direct Objects and Indirect Objects.**

50. D. *You* is a direct object and *with me* is a prepositional phrase. There is no indirect object. **Skill: Direct Objects and Indirect Objects.**

Section V. Biology

1. A. The first step in the scientific method is to state a question or problem based on an observation. The next step is to research and learn more about the topic from which the question originates. **Skill: An Introduction to Biology.**

2. A. Lipids are a class of biomolecules that provide a long-term storage solution for energy in living things. Examples of lipids include fats, steroids, and oils. **Skill: An Introduction to Biology.**

3. B. The purpose of a taxonomic system is to classify, describe, and name living things in an organized manner. **Skill: An Introduction to Biology.**

4. A. The control variable is a standard or constant that is used for comparisons. **Skill: An Introduction to Biology.**

5. B. To be catabolic, the glycolytic pathway must involve the breakdown of glucose into smaller molecules (called pyruvate) and the release of energy (in the form of ATP). **Skill: An Introduction to Biology.**

6. B. During anabolic metabolism, energy is absorbed as new substances like polymers are created. **Skill: An Introduction to Biology.**

7. A. The most basic unit and building block of all living things is the cell. **Skill: Cell Structure, Function, and Type.**

8. C. One characteristic of the cell theory is that cells arise from preexisting cells. This is the case for blood cells, which arise from stem progenitor cells. **Skill: Cell Structure, Function, and Type.**

9. C. The biological process of converting food sources into energy takes place in the mitochondria of the cell. Mitochondria are the cell's powerhouses that supply ATP (a form of energy) to the cell. **Skill: Cell Structure, Function, and Type.**

10. A. Organisms are classified as either autotrophs or heterotrophs according to how they obtain energy. Autotrophs obtain energy through sunlight, whereas heterotrophs obtain energy through food. **Skill: Cell Structure, Function, and Type.**

11. A. Only plant cells have cell walls, which help protect the cell and provide structural support. **Skill: Cell Structure, Function, and Type.**

12. D. Lysosomes are sac-like organelles that help keep the cell clean by breaking down substances such as worn out organelles and food. **Skill: Cell Structure, Function, and Type.**

13. A. Glycolysis involves the breakdown of glucose into pyruvate. Per one glucose molecule, this metabolic reaction yields a net of two molecules of ATP, two molecules of NADH, and two molecules of pyruvate. **Skill: Cellular Reproduction, Cellular Respiration, and Photosynthesis.**

14. A. Chiasmata are X-shaped structures that form when chromosomes from the mother and father of an organism undergoing meiosis are physically bound. This happens during prophase I of meiosis. **Skill: Cellular Reproduction, Cellular Respiration, and Photosynthesis.**

15. A. Plant cells build a new cell wall between the two daughter cells, while animal cells split by slowly pinching the cell membrane inward to divide the cell into two daughter cells. **Skill: Cellular Reproduction, Cellular Respiration, and Photosynthesis.**

16. C. After the first and second gap phases, DNA of the cell is replicated during the synthesis (or S) phase. **Skill: Cellular Reproduction, Cellular Respiration, and Photosynthesis.**

17. B. During the electron transport chain, chemiosmosis occurs. This happens when electrons and protons from NADH are released to generate large amounts of ATP. **Skill: Cellular Reproduction, Cellular Respiration, and Photosynthesis.**

18. B. A cell copies its DNA during the S phase, and nucleotides are the building blocks of DNA. Thus, the step preceding the S phase, the G_1 phase, is the phase of the cell cycle when the cell would contain the most nucleotides. **Skill: Cellular Reproduction, Cellular Respiration, and Photosynthesis.**

19. A. Diploid refers to the full number of chromosomes. **Skill: Genetics and DNA.**

20. B. After the DNA strand is separated, a complementary strand is assembled. **Skill: Genetics and DNA.**

21. B. Two of the offspring would be heterozygous tall (Ss), and the other two offspring would be homozygous short (ss). **Skill: Genetics and DNA.**

22. A. The RNA molecule is released into the cell for the next stage. **Skill: Genetics and DNA.**

23. D. Mendel developed theories of genetics that scientists around the world use today. **Skill: Genetics and DNA.**

24. A. The name of the factor used in Punnett squares is an allele. **Skill: Genetics and DNA.**

25. B. In eukaryotes, transcription produces pre-mRNA. **Skill: Genetics and DNA.**

Section VI. Chemistry

1. D. Around the world, the metric system is the accepted system of units for recording and communicating values. **Skill: Designing an Experiment.**

2. B. After a hypothesis is formed, variables are created when experiments are designed to test the hypothesis. **Skill: Designing an Experiment.**

3. B. The graph shows a non-correlation between height and birth month. This means birth month has no effect on how tall the baby will be. **Skill: Designing an Experiment.**

4. B. There is a positive correlation between weight and height. As weight increases, height also increases. This is shown by the graph's positive slope. **Skill: Designing an Experiment.**

5. C. Zinc-64 contains 30 protons and 34 neutrons. An isotope would contain the same number of protons but a different number of neutrons. **Skill: Scientific Notation.**

6. C. The nucleus has the largest mass because it contains multiple protons and neutrons, which have much more mass than the electrons in the electron cloud. **Skill: Scientific Notation.**

7. B. Because the exponent is negative, the decimal point moves to the left to convert to standard notation. After moving one space, it is on the other side of the 9. It moves 30 more spaces to the left, and the spaces are filled with zeros. **Skill: Scientific Notation.**

8. B. The exponent is negative 9, which means that the decimal point moves to the left nine spaces when converting to standard notation. **Skill: Scientific Notation.**

9. B. When converting a number to scientific notation, the coefficient must be between 1 and 10, which for this value would be 1.84. The exponent of positive 3 requires the decimal point to move three spaces to the right, which gives the correct value in standard notation. **Skill: Scientific Notation.**

10. D. The unit *g* stands for gram, which is a base unit of measure in the metric system. It is used to describe a unit value of mass for a given substance. **Skill: Temperature and the Metric System.**

11. C. Celsius and Fahrenheit are temperature scales that can be converted using the following formula: $C = \frac{5}{9}(F - 32)$. **Skill: Temperature and the Metric System.**

12. A. In the metric system, the multiplying factor used to convert 1 gram to a microgram is 10^{-6}. Thus, there is 0.000001 grams in a microgram. A gram is much larger than a microgram. **Skill: Temperature and the Metric System.**

13. D. The following formula is used to convert this value to Fahrenheit:

$$F = \left(\frac{9}{5}\right)C + 32$$

Where $F = \left(\frac{9}{5}\right) \times 110 + 32$. **Skill: Temperature and the Metric System.**

14. A. When a substance is boiling, liquid particles gain energy and move farther apart as they turn into gas. **Skill: States of Matter.**

15. D. At 100°C, all three halogens are gases. **Skill: States of Matter.**

16. C. Extensive properties deal with amounts, while intensive properties do not change based on amounts or other conditions. **Skill: Properties of Matter.**

17. C. Net water movement through a membrane in response to the concentration of a solute is called osmosis. **Skill: Properties of Matter.**

18. B. Basic substances turn litmus paper blue. Because KOH is a strong base, it will turn litmus blue. **Skill: Acids and Bases.**

19. C. As the water molecules are attracted to each other, which is cohesion, they also adhere to the sides of the xylem vessels, which transport water up to where it is needed in the plant. **Skill: Properties of Matter.**

20. C. Barium is a metal that could replace aluminum in a single-replacement reaction. The products for single-replacement reactions include an element (Al) that is replaced and a compound ($BaCl_2$). **Skill: Chemical Solutions.**

21. C. In a double-replacement reaction, two components, one from each reactant, change places. In this case, sodium and hydrogen replace each other. **Skill: Chemical Solutions.**

22. B. Because neither element involved is a metal, the bonds formed are covalent bonds, which means electrons are being shared. The Lewis structure shows silicon making four bonds to chlorine atoms. In each bond, two electrons are being shared for a total of eight shared electrons. **Skill: Chemical Bonds.**

23. C. In a chemical formula, the subscript after each element symbol shows the number of atoms of that element in one molecule. In methanol, there is one carbon atom, four hydrogen atoms, and one oxygen atom. **Skill: Chemical Bonds.**

24. B. In the graph, the line for 30 grams of solute crosses the line for $KClO_3$ at 70°C. **Skill: Chemical Solutions.**

25. D. A weak acid is a substance that has a pH value less than 7. Salmon has an estimated pH of 6, so it is most likely a weak acid. **Skill: Acids and Bases.**

Section VII. Anatomy & Physiology

1. B. This is a negative feedback mechanism because its goal is to readjust the internal environment to return it to a steady, constant, healthy state. **Skill: Organization of the Human Body.**

2. A. Connective tissue includes cells of the immune system and cells of the blood. **Skill: Organization of the Human Body.**

3. D. As blood flows out of the right atrium into the right ventricle, the tricuspid valve prevents blood from flowing back into the right atrium. **Skill: Cardiovascular System.**

4. C. Thrombocytes, erythrocytes, and leukocytes are formed elements found in blood. Erythocytes are the smallest with a cell diameter of 0.008 millimeters, while leukocytes are the largest with a cell diameter of 0.02 millimeters. **Skill: Cardiovascular System.**

5. **D.** The trachea is a hollow tube in the upper respiratory tract that branches off into bronchi, which extend into the lungs. **Skill: The Respiratory System.**

6. **B.** The larynx is also referred to as the voice box because the vocal cords are housed there. **Skill: The Respiratory System.**

7. **D.** Sucrase is the enzyme that breaks down sucrose. **Skill: Gastrointestinal System.**

8. **A.** The correct sequence of the four parts of the large intestine is ascending, transverse, descending, and sigmoid. **Skill: Gastrointestinal System.**

9. **B.** Pregnancy typically lasts for about 40 weeks, which are traditionally divided into three periods of about 13 weeks each called trimesters. **Skill: Reproductive System.**

10. **D.** The ovaries and testes produce female and male gametes, respectively, and are analogs. **Skill: Reproductive System.**

11. **A.** During macroscopic urinalysis, a medical professional visually observes differences in a urine sample. Additionally, the medical professional can analyze for the presence of certain substances, at specific concentrations, by using urinary dipsticks. The dipstick must change color and be compared to a standard chart to confirm something about the urine. **Skill: The Urinary System.**

12. **A.** Urine is a byproduct of the blood that is filtered in the kidneys. This tubular filtrate travels to the ureter, which is a muscular tube that contracts to push urine to the urethra and out of the body. **Skill: The Urinary System.**

13. **D.** Within compact bone are several units called osteons. These osteons have a canal running through them called the Haversian canal. This canal contains the blood vessels and nerve fibers in bone. **Skill: Skeletal System.**

14. **C.** Osteoclasts are bone-resorbing cells that break down bone. Osteoblasts are bone cells that aid in bone formation. Working together, these bone cells facilitate a process called bone remodeling. **Skill: Skeletal System.**

15. **D.** All muscles have the ability to contract and extend. To work together, all muscles contract (or shorten) and extend (or lengthen) in pairs following stimulation from the nervous system. **Skill: Muscular System.**

16. **C.** Cardiac muscle is a striated, branched type of muscle found only in the heart. Cardiac muscle is under involuntary control. **Skill: Muscular System.**

17. **C.** The hair shaft is the portion of hair found on the surface of the body. It is not attached to the hair follicle, which is in the dermis. **Skill: Integumentary System.**

18. **D.** The stratum spinosum contains keratinocytes, which are affected by squamous cell carcinoma. This skin layer is part of the epidermis. **Skill: Integumentary System.**

19. A. Epidermal cells are found deep in the stratum basale. From there, they travel to the skin's surface, producing keratin along the way. This keratin creates the waterproof layer, or stratum corneum. **Skill: Integumentary System.**

20. C. The cell body, or soma, contains the nucleus of the neuron. Inside the nucleus is DNA, which contains the genetic information for the neuron. Other organelles are also found inside the cell body. **Skill: The Nervous System.**

21. A. The nervous system controls many parts of the body by coordinating activities. Its primary function with help from the endocrine system is to maintain homeostasis. **Skill: The Nervous System.**

22. C. Paracrine chemical signals are released by cells and have effects on other cell types. Somatostatin, secreted by the pancreas, inhibits the release of insulin by other cells in the pancreas. **Skill: Endocrine System.**

23. C. The term *ductless* indicates that hormones are secreted directly into the blood. **Skill: Endocrine System.**

24. C. The mucous covering the respiratory membranes is the first line of defense in the lymphatic system. **Skill: The Lymphatic System.**

25. C. The thymus gland secretes hormones that stimulate the maturation of the killer T cells. It is active from birth through puberty. **Skill: The Lymphatic System.**

Section VIII. Physics

1. D. A ball thrown into the air undergoes projectile motion once released. The shape of the path it follows is a parabola (that is, the path is parabolic). **Skill: Nature of Motion.**

2. B. If two vectors have the same length but opposite directions, adding them yields 0. One way to understand this is to call a the length of $\vec{x}$ and $\vec{u}$ the unit vector in the direction of $\vec{x}$. Then, $\vec{x} = a\vec{u}$ and, therefore, $\vec{y} = -a\vec{u}$. Their sum is 0. **Skill: Nature of Motion.**

3. C. The standard form of a vector is the head coordinates minus the tail coordinates. In this case, the head coordinates are unknown. Start by writing an expression for the vector. Let the head coordinates be (x, y), for example.

$(2, 6) = (x - 3, y - 1)$

Solve the two equations for x and y:

$x - 3 = 2$

$x = 5$

$y - 1 = 6$

$y = 7$

Skill: Nature of Motion.

4. B. To find the force in the direction of a certain vector, first divide that vector by its length to get a unit vector. The length of (1.0, 2.0) is 2.2.

$$\frac{1}{2.2}(1.0, 2.0) = \left(0.45, 0.91\right)$$

Next, multiply by the magnitude of the force in newtons.

$$3.5 \times (0.45, 0.91) = \left(1.6, 3.2\right)$$

Skill: Nature of Motion.

5. B. The speed, if constant, is equal to the distance divided by the travel time. Therefore, the travel time is the distance divided by the speed:

$$\frac{490 \; miles}{65 \; miles \; per \; hour} = 7.5 \; hours$$

Skill: Nature of Motion.

6. B. When a player throws a ball, it will (under ideal conditions with no friction) undergo projectile motion, following a parabola. That motion is neither linear nor rotational; the best description in this case is nonlinear. **Skill: Friction.**

7. D. If a planet has a nonzero speed and is a constant distance from a star, it must be moving in a circular orbit. Although that motion is nonlinear, the most descriptive term is *rotational*. **Skill: Friction.**

8. A. Draw a circle and mark the rightmost point as the location of the car. If north is up, then the centripetal acceleration of the car will be west—that is, to the left. Next, mark the leftmost point on the circle: this is the location of the car after it has gone halfway around the circle. Because the centripetal acceleration is always toward the center of circular motion, it will be east—that is, to the right. **Skill: Friction.**

9. B. The centrifugal force, which is a "ghost force," is the feeling of being pushed in a certain direction when undergoing rotational motion. The centripetal force, which is a real force, is always in the opposite direction. Thus, if the pilot feels an upward force, the centripetal force must be downward, making answer B correct. **Skill: Friction.**

10 C. The angular frequency ω is $\frac{2\pi}{T}$, where T is the period. Thus,

$$T = \frac{2\pi}{\omega}$$

The velocity is the circumference of the circle ($2\pi r$) divided by the period.

$$v = \frac{2\pi r}{T} = \frac{2\pi r}{2\pi/\omega} = r\omega = (42 \; m)(0.29 \; Hz) = 12 \; m/s$$

Skill: Friction.

11. A. Both electromagnetic and mechanical waves can travel through materials and exhibit refraction. They also both obey the wave-speed equation. By elimination, only electromagnetic waves can exist in a vacuum. (As their name indicates, mechanical waves require some material—solid, liquid, or gas—to propagate.) **Skill: Waves and Sounds.**

12. B. Two atoms are the same element if they have the same number of protons. Only choice B fits this definition. **Skill: Waves and Sounds.**

13. D. Because c is the maximum speed of light, the wave speed must (under normal conditions) be less than or equal to c. Because the wave speed is related to the index of refraction by $v = c/n$, n must be greater than or equal to 1 to prevent v from exceeding c. **Skill: Waves and Sounds.**

14. B. If two isotopes are of the same element, they have the same number of protons but different numbers of neutrons (and, therefore, different numbers of nucleons). Because one is charged and one is neutral, one must have more electrons than the other. **Skill: Waves and Sounds.**

15. A. Like charges repel, so if the experimenter knows the charge polarity of one object (positive), he knows that the other object has the same charge polarity if they exert a repulsive force on each other. **Skill: Waves and Sounds.**

16. D. When velocity is zero, impulse, momentum, and kinetic energy are zero. However, a stationary object could have a height above ground and therefore possess potential energy. **Skill: Kinetic Energy.**

17. B. The kinetic energy is 4 times greater because during free-fall all potential energy is converted to kinetic energy (ignoring wind resistance), and the potential energy is directly related to the height. **Skill: Kinetic Energy.**

18. D. The bell has stored energy. This energy is potential due to the bell's height above ground. **Skill: Kinetic Energy.**

19. B. Because velocity is squared in the kinetic energy formula, a change in velocity by a factor of 2 results in a change in kinetic energy by a factor of 4. **Skill: Kinetic Energy.**

20. A. The mass is directly proportional to the force. **Skill: Kinetic Energy.**

21. C. A field line describes the path a (positive) test charge would follow if placed somewhere around a given charge configuration. Because positive charge repels positive and negative charge attracts positive, a test charge will be repelled by the positive charge and attracted to the negative charge. Therefore, the field lines will originate from the positive charge and end at the negative charge. **Skill: Electricity and Magnetism.**

22. C. Electromagnetic induction—the creation of an electric force in a conductor (a wire loop, in this case)—is the result of changing magnetic flux inside the loop. **Skill: Electricity and Magnetism.**

23. C. The field at a given point is the force that would be exerted on a 1-coulomb "test charge" placed there. In this case, because the force on a 1-coulomb charge is known, the field strength is the same value (albeit with different units). **Skill: Electricity and Magnetism.**

24. A. Because the electrons are equidistant from the proton, the forces they exert on the proton are equal in magnitude (both are attractive forces). But because these particles lie on a line, the forces have opposite directions, so they cancel each other out. **Skill: Electricity and Magnetism.**

25. B. Use Coulomb's law, noting that the field is the force on a 1-coulomb test charge. Alternatively, use the field formula:

$$E = k\frac{Q}{r^2}$$

$$E = \left(9 \times 10^9\right)\frac{5.0 \times 10^{-3}}{(3.0 \times 10^2)^2}$$

$$E = (9 \times 10^9)\frac{5.0 \times 10^{-3}}{9.0 \times 10^4} = 5.0 \times 10^2 \; newtons\; per\; coulomb$$

Skill: Electricity and Magnetism.

HESI PRACTICE EXAM 3

SECTION I. MATHEMATICS

You have 50 minutes to complete 50 questions.

1. **What is $4 + 5 + 12 + 9$?**
    - A. 20
    - B. 30
    - C. 40
    - D. 50

2. **What is the difference between two equal numbers?**
    - A. Negative
    - B. Positive
    - C. Zero
    - D. Not enough information

3. **What is the difference between two negative numbers?**
    - A. Negative number
    - B. Positive number
    - C. Zero
    - D. Not enough information

4. **Kevin has 120 minutes to complete an exam. If he is already used 43, how many minutes does he have left?**
    - A. 43
    - B. 77
    - C. 87
    - D. 163

5. **Evaluate the expression $154 + 98$.**
    - A. 250
    - B. 252
    - C. 352
    - D. 15,498

6. **What is $762 \div 127$?**
    - A. 4
    - B. 6
    - C. 8
    - D. 9

7. **Evaluate the expression $3 + 1 - 5 + 2 - 6$.**
    - A. −9
    - B. −5
    - C. 0
    - D. 17

8. **What is $1,566 \div 54$?**
    - A. 2755
    - B. 28
    - C. 29
    - D. 1,512

9. **Evaluate the expression $6 + (1 - (2 + (5 - (3 - 1))))$.**
    - A. −2
    - B. 2
    - C. 6
    - D. 18

10. **Which statement about multiplication and division is true?**
    - A. The product of the quotient and the dividend is the divisor.
    - B. The product of the dividend and the divisor is the quotient.
    - C. The product of the quotient and the divisor is the dividend.
    - D. None of the above.

11. **Which decimal is the least?**
    - A. 2.22
    - B. 2.02
    - C. 2.002
    - D. 2.2

12. **Which fraction is the least?**
    - A. $\frac{5}{6}$
    - B. $\frac{3}{4}$
    - C. $\frac{17}{24}$
    - D. $\frac{2}{3}$

13. **Write 290% as a fraction.**
    - A. $2\frac{9}{200}$
    - B. $2\frac{9}{100}$
    - C. $2\frac{9}{20}$
    - D. $2\frac{9}{10}$

14. Which fraction is the greatest?

   A. $\frac{3}{10}$　　　C. $\frac{1}{2}$

   B. $\frac{2}{5}$　　　D. $\frac{1}{4}$

15. Multiply $3\frac{1}{5} \times \frac{5}{8}$.

   A. 1　　　C. 3

   B. 2　　　D. 4

16. Multiply $2 \times \frac{3}{4}$.

   A. $\frac{1}{4}$　　　C. $1\frac{1}{2}$

   B. $\frac{3}{8}$　　　D. $2\frac{3}{4}$

17. Divide $8 \div \frac{2}{9}$.

   A. 9　　　C. 36

   B. 18　　　D. 72

18. Multiply $\frac{2}{5} \times 3$.

   A. $\frac{2}{15}$　　　C. $2\frac{3}{5}$

   B. $1\frac{1}{5}$　　　D. $3\frac{2}{5}$

19. If a survey finds that 120 people are in group X and 230 people are in group Y, what is the ratio of people in group Y to people in group X or group Y?

   A. 12:35　　　C. 23:35

   B. 12:23　　　D. 35:23

20. If a company's automobile fleet includes 132 cars of brand A and 48 cars of brand B, what is the fleet's ratio of brand B to brand A?

   A. 4:11　　　C. 15:11

   B. 11:15　　　D. 11:4

21. Which expression is different from the others?

   A. 2:5　　　C. 40%

   B. $\frac{2}{5}$　　　D. 0.04

22. What is 36% as a ratio?

   A. 9:25　　　C. 18:40

   B. 36:100　　　D. 25:9

23. If the population of an endangered frog species fell from 2,250 individuals to 2,115 individuals in a year, what is that population's annual rate of increase?

   A. −135%　　　C. 6%

   B. −6%　　　D. 135%

24. Convert 99 meters to kilometers.

   A. 0.0099 kilometers

   B. 0.099 kilometers

   C. 0.9 kilometers

   D. 9.9 kilometers

25. Identify 3:00 p.m. in military time.

   A. 0300　　　C. 1200

   B. 0600　　　D. 1500

26. Identify 1920 in 12-hour clock time.

   A. 6:20 p.m.　　　C. 6:20 a.m.

   B. 7:20 p.m.　　　D. 7:20 a.m.

27. Convert 10 quarts to fluid ounces.

   A. 20 fluid ounces　　　C. 200 fluid ounces

   B. 32 fluid ounces　　　D. 320 fluid ounces

28. Convert 4,388 decimeters to meters.

   A. 438.8 meters　　　C. 4.388 meters

   B. 43.88 meters　　　D. 0.4388 meters

29. Solve the equation for the unknown, $\frac{x}{2} + 5 = 8$.

   A. $\frac{3}{2}$　　　C. 6

   B. $\frac{5}{2}$　　　D. 26

30. Solve the inequality for the unknown,
$\frac{1}{4}(3-x) + x + 1 < \frac{1}{2}(2-x)$.

  A. $x < -1$

  B. $x > -1$

  C. $x < -\frac{3}{5}$

  D. $x > -\frac{3}{5}$

31. Solve the equation for the unknown,
$3x + 8 = 12$.

  A. $\frac{3}{4}$

  B. 1

  C. $\frac{4}{3}$

  D. 2

32. Solve the inequality for the unknown,
$3x + 5 - 2(x + 3) > 4(1-x) + 5$.

  A. $x > 2$

  B. $x > 9$

  C. $x > 10$

  D. $x > 17$

33. Solve the system of equations,
$2y + x = -20$
$y = -x - 12$.

  A. (4, 8)

  B. (4, -8)

  C. (-4, 8)

  D. (-4, -8)

34. Solve the system of equations, $\begin{matrix} y = -x \\ x^2 + y^2 = 8 \end{matrix}$.

  A. (1, 1) and (-1, -1)

  B. (1, -1) and (-1, 1)

  C. (2, 2) and (-2, -2)

  D. (2, -2) and (-2, 2)

35. Solve the system of equations,
$y = -2x + 3$
$y + x = 5$.

  A. (-2, 7)   C. (2, -7)

  B. (-2, -7)   D. (2, 7)

36. Solve the system of equations by graphing, $\begin{array}{l} 3x + y = -1 \\ 2x - y = -4 \end{array}$.

A.

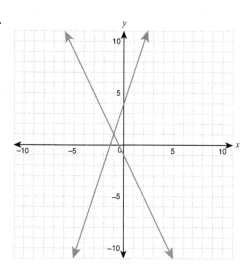

C.

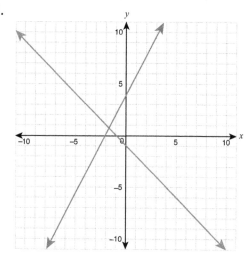

B.

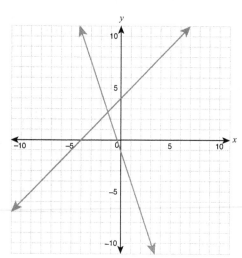

D.

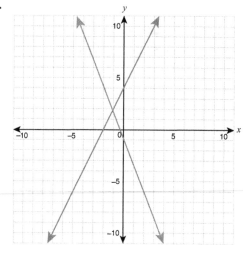

37. Solve the system of equations by graphing, $\begin{array}{l} y = -x + 7 \\ y = 2x - 8 \end{array}$.

A.

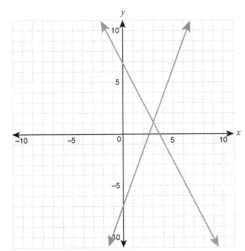

C.

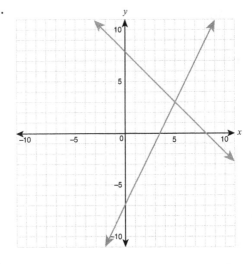

B.

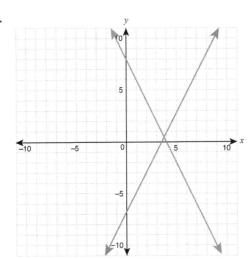

D.

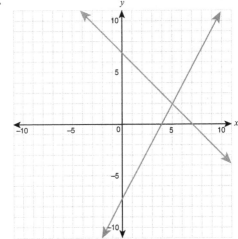

38. Eric buys $2\frac{2}{5}$ pounds of apples each week for four weeks. How many total pounds does he buy?

A. $7\frac{3}{5}$ C. $9\frac{3}{5}$

B. $8\frac{2}{5}$ D. $10\frac{2}{5}$

39. An even roll of a number cube results in +2 points, and an odd roll of a number cube is –3 points. If there are 14 even numbers and 11 odd numbers, then how many points are scored?

A. –61 C. 5

B. –5 D. 61

40. A person has $250 in a checking account and writes checks for $70, $85, $60, and $100. There is also a fee of $20. What is the balance of the account?

A. –$335 C. $335

B. –$85 D. $685

41. A teacher buys 4 bottles of water for class. Each bottle of water contains 3 liters. Each cup holds $\frac{2}{5}$ of a liter. How many cups can be filled?

A. 12 C. 42

B. 30 D. 60

42. One online seller has about 6×10^8 online orders, and another online seller has about 5×10^7 online orders. How many times more orders does the first company have?

   A. 12   C. 20

   B. 15   D. 32

43. Simplify $\left(\frac{x^0}{y^{-2}}\right)^2$.

   A. $\frac{1}{y^4}$ C. y^4

   B. $\frac{x}{y^4}$ D. $x^4 y^4$

44. A lysosome has a length of 1×10^{-6} meter, and measles virus has a length of 2×10^{-9} meter. How many times longer is the lysosome?

   A. 5   C. 500

   B. 50   D. 5,000

45. Simplify $\left(\frac{x^5}{5}\right)^4$.

   A. $\frac{x^9}{20}$ C. $\frac{x^{20}}{20}$

   B. $\frac{x^{20}}{625}$ D. $\frac{x^9}{625}$

46. Solve $x^2 = 169$.

   A. $-10, 10$ C. $-12, 12$

   B. $-11, 11$ D. $-13, 13$

47. Multiply, $(4x + 5)(3x-2)$.

   A. $12x^2-7x + 10$ C. $12x^2 + 7x-10$

   B. $12x^2 + 7x + 10$ D. $12x^2-7x-10$

48. Apply the polynomial identity to rewrite $27x^3-8$.

   A. $(3x-2)(9x^2-6x + 4)$

   B. $(3x-2)(9x^2 + 6x + 4)$

   C. $(3x-2)(9x^2 + 6x-4)$

   D. $(3x-2)(9x^2-6x-4)$

49. Perform the operation,

   $(-2x^2 + 8x) + (3x^3-4x^2 + 1)$.

   A. $3x^3-6x^2 + 8x + 1$

   B. $3x^3-2x^2 + 8x + 1$

   C. $3x^3 + 6x^2 + 8x + 1$

   D. $3x^3 + 2x^2 + 8x + 1$

50. Apply the polynomial identity to rewrite $16x^2-121$.

   A. $(x + 11)(x-11)$ C. $(4x + 11)(4x-11)$

   B. $(x-11)^2$ D. $(4x-11)^2$

SECTION II. READING COMPREHENSION

You have 50 minutes to complete 47 questions.

Please read the text below and answer questions 1-5.

Desserts are known as the "forbidden food" in most diets. But dark chocolate is a sweet that people can enjoy because of its undeniable health benefits. Categorized as an "antioxidant," dark chocolate is known to fight free radicals, the unbalanced compounds created by cellular processes that can harm the body. This amazing sweet treat is also known to lower blood pressure, improve blood flow, and reduce heart disease risk in people. Studies have shown that dark chocolate can even improve people's brain function. There is considerable evidence that dark chocolate can provide powerful benefits, but it is still loaded with calories, so consuming too much is not recommended. People can reap the benefits of dark chocolate by eating it in moderation.

1. **The topic of this paragraph is:**

    A. foods that battle heart disease.

    B. healthy dessert recipes.

    C. cooking with dark chocolate.

    D. benefits of dark chocolate.

2. **The topic sentence of this paragraph is:**

    A. Desserts are known as the "forbidden food" in most diets.

    B. But dark chocolate is a sweet that people can enjoy because of its undeniable health benefits.

    C. This amazing sweet treat is also know to lower blood pressure, improve blood flow, and reduce heart disease risk in people.

    D. People can reap the benefits of dark chocolate by eating it in moderation.

3. **If the author added a description of a popular recipe using dark chocolate as its main ingredient, what type of information would this be?**

    A. A main idea

    B. A topic sentence

    C. A supporting detail

    D. An off-topic sentence

4. **Read the following description of the paragraph:**

The author fails to offer a holistic view of dark chocolate by only presenting its benefits and never exploring its downsides.

Why is this not a valid description of the main idea?

A. It is not accurate; the author of the paragraph is stating facts, not opinions.

B. It is not objective; the person summarizing the main idea is biased since he/she is in the medical field.

C. It is not accurate; the author of the paragraph does warn the reader to eat dark chocolate in moderation.

D. It is not objective; the person summarizing the main idea is obviously not a fan of dark chocolate.

5. **Why isn't a statistic about how much chocolate is consumed on a daily basis by the average American suitable for this passage?**

A. It does not directly support the main idea that dark chocolate is good for your health.

B. Readers might feel the author is passing judgment on how much chocolate Americans consume.

C. Statistics should never be used as supporting details in persuasive writing.

D. It would act as a second topic sentence and confuse readers about the main idea.

Read the following sentence and answer questions 6-8.

Studies conducted on numerous kindergarten programs across the country have revealed eye-opening evidence that today's kindergarten curriculum looks more like the curriculum taught in first grade classrooms thirty years ago.

6. **What is the main idea of the above sentence?**

A. What kindergarten is

B. How kindergarten has changed

C. What students learn in kindergarten

D. What the kindergarten curriculum is

7. **Imagine this sentence is a *supporting detail* in a well-developed paragraph. Which of the following sentences would best function as a *topic sentence*?**

A. The curriculum seen in today's kindergarten classrooms may not be developmentally appropriate for children.

B. Teaching styles have changed dramatically over the course of the last thirty years.

C. Play-based learning is still a big part of today's kindergarten classrooms.

D. Studies have shown that national-based standards lead to more success in the classroom.

8. Imagine this sentence is the *topic sentence* of a well-developed paragraph. Which of the following sentences would best function as a *supporting detail*?

A. Some students enter kindergarten with a rich nursery school experience while others enter the school environment for the first time in their lives.

B. Kindergarten is a German word that literally means "a garden for children."

C. While kindergarteners from years ago only needed to begin to learn basic concepts of print in reading, today's kindergarteners are expected to be at an E reading level when leaving the classroom.

D. Kindergarten is the time when children acquire the necessary early educational skills to prepare them to be full-fledged students who are ready for first grade.

9. A summary is a _____.

A. retelling of all the ideas of a text

B. review of the final idea of a text

C. rundown of the first idea of a text

D. restatement of the main ideas of a text

10. Which graphic would you use to show a sequence of decisions involved in a complex process?

A. Diagram   C. Bar graph

B. Flowchart   D. Pie chart

11. Which graphic would you use to convey the differences between numerical values using rectangles?

A. Diagram   C. Bar Graph

B. Flowchart   D. Pie Chart

12. Which of the following would make a summary ineffective?

A. One that is objective

B. One that uses new words

C. One full of the main ideas

D. One that is structurally plagiarized

Read the following text and then answer questions 13-15.

In the late morning, Cynthia met Max at the state park where he had been waiting. They went on a hike. They followed a path that first led them through the deep, lush woods. The path then took them past a beautiful, serene lake. They were beginning to get thirsty, so they stopped to sit on a large rock to drink some water. Next, they continued hiking and came upon a clearing, Cynthia was astonished to see a picnic blanket all set up with plates and a picnic basket.

"Max!" she exclaimed.

Max had set up the picnic to surprise Cynthia.

13. According to the paragraph, which event happened first?

A. Cynthia met Max at a state park in the late morning.

B. Max set up the picnic for him and Cynthia.

C. Cynthia and Max walked past a lake.

D. Cynthia and Max stopped to drink water on a rock.

14. **Which word clues help you understand that this event happened first?**

    A. "had set up"

    B. "first went"

    C. "beginning to get"

    D. "in the late morning"

15. **Which of the following words from the passage is *not* a sequence word?**

    A. First   C. Next

    B. Then   D. Beginning

16. **Read the sentences below.**

    Simon decided to play football all day instead of study for his math test. He received a poor grade.

    Which word or phrase, if inserted at the beginning of sentence two, would effectively transition between these two ideas?

    A. Likewise   C. As a result

    B. However   D. For example

Read the passage below and answer questions 17-23.

When my 13-year-old daughter entered the house, the door slammed open with a celebratory "bang!" I was instantly dismayed to see that my first-born stomped right by me as I held my arms open for a warm hug.

"How was your day, honey?" I asked as she gave me her quintessential eye roll.

I sat across from her ready to hear how marvelous her day was. However, I only got an earful of all the drama that had ensued at school: "So-and-so said this,"

"gym was a drag," "Mr. Fletcher doesn't like me because I am not a math genius."

My head ached from nodding so much, so I got up quickly to bring her something.

"Mom! How could you get up when I'm in the middle of telling you about my life?" she barked.

Despite her protest, her eyes could not help but light up when I brought her a freshly baked chocolate chip cookie on a plate.

I guess life isn't all that bad, is it?

17. **Which adjectives best describe the tone of the passage?**

    A. Ironic, furious

    B. Honest, furious

    C. Ironic, amusing

    D. Honest, amusing

18. **Which sentence from the passage is clearly ironic?**

    A. "How was your day, honey?"

    B. I sat across from her ready to hear how marvelous her day was.

    C. My head ached from nodding so much, so I got up quickly to bring her something.

    D. "Mom! How could you get up when I'm in the middle of telling you about my life?"

19. The author of the passage first establishes the ironic tone by:

   A. describing the slamming of the door as "celebratory."

   B. quoting the daughter's words.

   C. explaining how the mother got up to get the daughter cookie.

   D. having the mother state that life "isn't all that bad."

20. Reread the following sentence:

   I guess life isn't all that bad, is it?

   Which adjective could describe an effective reader's mood when reading this line in the context of the passage?

   A. Entertained   C. Empathetic

   B. Frustrated   D. Dismissive

21. **Which word or phrase does *not* function as a transition in the passage?**

   A. Instantly   C. So

   B. However   D. Despite

22. The transitions "however" and "despite" link ideas in the passage by showing:

   A. when events happen in time.

   B. how certain ideas contrast.

   C. examples that illustrate ideas.

   D. cause-and-effect relationships.

23. Reread the following sentence:

   "How was your day, honey?" I asked as she gave me her quintessential eye roll.

   Which transition would you use if the next sentence describes the daughter *also* making a "tsk" sound to show her frustration?

   A. Finally   C. To illustrate

   B. Furthermore   D. Nevertheless

24. The author's _____ is his or her general outlook or set of opinions about the subject.

   A. purpose   C. main idea

   B. reasoning   D. point of view

Read the following text and answer questions 25-28.

Our survey revealed some eye-opening results about young people and the role technology plays in their lives: technology is the primary focus of young people today. In our survey, 85% of those questioned said they spend their free time using technology in some way. Only 5% claim that they read actual books, 7% hang out with friends, and only 3% do some sort of physical activity. Whether it's looking through social media sites, playing video games, texting friends, or surfing the web, our youth spends an inordinate amount of time on screens. The days of hanging with friends, being outside in nature, and reading a good book for fun seem to be long gone.

Natalie Greenburg, clinical psychologist from the Perkins Institute, claims that, "Studies have shown a direct correlation between too much screen time and rising depression rates among teens." Greenburg explains screen time has an impact on how individuals view themselves. This is based on the amount of likes someone gets on social media sites or the number of texts someone receives from his or her peers. "The feedback kids get from technology becomes the barometer for their self-worth, which could lead to depression." Cyber bullying is also a big issue with technology. "Kids are able to freely say anything they want behind a screen," Greenburg states, "Since they are bullying from a keyboard, kids are no longer exposed to social cues like facial expressions and body language, which may stop the behavior. As a result, cyber bullying has become rampant, which has led to more depression."

Technology is here to stay and it is only going to become more entrenched in our society. It will continue to impact our youth in ways we can't even fathom.

25. What is the primary purpose of the passage?

A. To inform
C. To persuade

B. To caution
D. To entertain

26. With which statement would the author of the passage most likely agree with?

A. Technology is having a negative impact on our youth.

B. Technology will become eventually become obsolete.

C. Technology will change for the better in the near future.

D. Technology provides our youth with endless possibilities.

27. Which sentence would express an additional effective reason to support the main idea of this passage?

A. Every teacher feels technology is getting in the way of classroom learning.

B. A recent screen time study shows that technology use has risen since it is available in so many forms.

C. Everyone feels young people have no hope since they are too dependent on technology.

D. All young people know they are more technologically savvy than their parents will ever be.

28. The author most likely included Natalie Greenburg's comments in order to:

A. explain the effects that technology is having on young people.

B. add an emotional component to the statistical information presented.

C. appeal to the reader's reason by adding statistical data to back up an opinion.

D. distract readers by tricking them into believing the argument is not sufficiently supported.

Read the following text and answer questions 29-31.

As Time Goes On is a painfully realistic depiction of what life is like for some senior citizens in the twilight of their lives. Tabitha Reynolds artfully captures the harsh reality people face when they grow old. From one's physical limitations to the emotional toll of letting go of one's former self, Reynolds pays homage to this fragile yet meaningful time in a person's life.

The book chronicles the final years of Audrey Lacoste's life. A former prima ballerina, Audrey is now a prisoner to her rheumatoid arthritis. The disease has limited Audrey's body in ways she could never have imagined. Her physical ailment coupled with the loss of her beloved husband causes her two self-involved children to move her into *Sunshine Cove*, an assisted living facility. The facility is anything but sunny, but slowly the light in Audrey's life begins to flicker once again when she makes an unexpected friend.

A New York Times best seller for seven consecutive weeks, *As Time Goes On* is a must read. The words will make you laugh, cry, gasp and sigh as you travel along the rocky road to the end of Audrey's life.

29. The purpose of this passage is to:

    A. decide.   C. persuade.
    B. inform.   D. entertain.

30. Which detail from the passage is factual?

    A. *As Time Goes On* is a painfully realistic depiction of what life is like for some senior citizens...

    B. Tabitha Reynolds artfully captures the harsh reality people face as they grow old.

    C. The book chronicles the final years of Audrey Lacoste's life.

    D. ...*As Time Goes On* is a must read.

31. The author of the passage includes details about Audrey Lacoste's life in order to appeal to the reader's:

    A. reason.   C. feelings.
    B. trust.   D. knowledge.

32. Which of the following is an opinion?

    A. Doctors should offer holistic approaches instead of relying solely on medication.

    B. Non-steroidal anti-inflammatory drugs are the most prescribed medications by doctors.

    C. Pharmaceutical companies spend double the amount on marketing to doctors than they spend on research.

    D. A 2018 study predicts that the U.S. will experience a shortage of between 42,600 and 121,300 physicians by 2030.

33. Which of the following is a form of faulty reasoning?

    A. An overgeneralization

    B. A statement of opinion

    C. A documented statistic

    D. A verifiable piece of information

34. Which statement, if true, is a fact?

   A. The 2018 London New Year's Day Parade had more spectators than the 2018 NFL Super Bowl.

   B. The 2018 London New Year's Day Parade was more exciting than the 2018 NFL Super Bowl.

   C. The 2018 London New Year's Day Parade was a fantastic display of award-winning marching bands, creatively designed parade floats, and international celebrities.

   D. The 2018 London New Year's Day Parade caused greater joy and entertainment than the 2018 NFL Super Bowl.

Read the following passage and answer questions 35-38.

Working mothers are required to perform a balancing act between their work and home lives every day or else everything will fall apart. Not only do they have mounds of work responsibilities, but also are expected to be the primary caregiver as well as the cook, cleaner, and organizer at home. Even though times have changed and more fathers are involved in parenting and home duties, the onus ultimately still falls on the working mother. Working mothers are shortchanged because they rarely get the chance to sit back and allow someone else to assume their responsibilities.

35. What is the primary argument in the passage?

   A. Working mothers have it hard.

   B. More mothers have entered the workforce.

   C. Fathers today are more willing to pitch in at home.

   D. Working mothers cannot survive without the help of fathers.

36. What assumption in this passage reflects negative stereotypical thinking?

   A. Fathers have jobs just like mothers do.

   B. A lot of mothers today have full-time jobs.

   C. Today's fathers are more involved at home.

   D. Mothers cook, clean, and care for the children.

37. The argument in the pragraph is invalid because the author:

   A. suggests that working mothers choose to have such hectic lives.

   B. uses derogatory and disrespectful language to describe fathers.

   C. describes working mothers in a negative way that makes it seem as though they only look out for themselves.

   D. professes an interest in all that working mothers do while simultaneously suggesting that fathers don't do enough.

38. **Re-read the following sentence from the passage:**

Working mothers are required to perform a balancing act between their work and home lives every day or else everything will fall apart.

What type of faulty reasoning does this sentence display?

A. Either/or fallacy

B. Circular reasoning

C. Bandwagon argument

D. False statement of cause and effect

39. _____ provide information that is simplified or highly summarized.

A. Primary sources

B. Secondary sources

C. Tertiary sources

D. Quaternary sources

40. **Which of the following is an example of a secondary source?**

A. A diary of a politician

B. A biography of a politician

C. A study guide on a politician's speech

D. An encyclopedia article about a politician

41. **Which of the following sources should be treated with skepticism even though it is primary?**

A. The field notes of a scientist studying primate behavior in the wild

B. A diary of a child who operated a loom in the Lowell Mills

C. An interview with a ninety-two-year-old Holocaust survivor

D. An article from the turn of the 19ᵗʰ century about the best farming practices

Read the following passage and answer questions 42-44.

Manny looked out the window.

"Not yet," he mumbled to himself.

He walked into the kitchen to try to distract himself. He was about to open the cookie jar when he heard a car motor.

"Now?" he ran to the window.

"Ugh," he sighed, "it is just Mr. Mendez."

Suddenly he saw it. The small, white truck he was searching for.

He burst through the door and breathlessly greeted Stanley.

Stanley smiled as he handed a stack of envelopes to Manny.

"Is this what you're looking for, son?" Stanley said with a smile.

Manny looked at the return address. *Michigan State University*.

"Yes! Thank you!" Manny cried as he bolted into his house.

"Good luck, Manny!" Stanley yelled after him.

42. **From the text above, you can infer that Manny is:**

A. best friends with Stanley.

B. anxiously awaiting the mail.

C. very hard on himself.

D. not a fan of Mr. Mendez.

43. **Which detail does *not* provide evidence to back up the conclusion that Manny is eager for the mail to come?**

A. He mumbles "not yet" to himself.

B. He is about to open the cookie jar.

C. He sighs when he sees Mr. Mendez.

D. He bursts through the door and greets Stanley.

44. **Which detail from the text supports the inference that Stanley knows Manny pretty well?**

A. He drives up in his truck.

B. He hands him a stack of envelopes.

C. He asks if an envelope is what he is looking for.

D. He smiles at Manny.

Read the following passage and answer questions 45-47.

Are you tired of your children not listening to you? Do they seem distracted every time you ask them to do something? Are you met with a glossy-eyed stare every time you say something to them? Part of the problem is too much screen time.

Technology has its benefits, but it does a lot to ruin our children's focus. There are too many flashes of light, too many colors, too many hyperlinks to navigate – it's a wonder our children can even focus at all!

Limiting your children's screen time would do wonders for them. Make more time to have face-to-face conversations. This will allow your children to actually practice good listening *and* communication skills. Hand them a book! This will help them sit still and focus on *one* thing for a period of time.

Technology won't be going away anytime soon, but you can set limits for your children to help them focus, listen, and better engage with you.

45. **This article is written for:**

    A. parents   C. teachers

    B. children   D. policymakers

46. **The author of this article assumes that:**

    A. parents are frustrated by their children not listening to them.

    B. parents are on screens more than their children are.

    C. children do not like to be told what to do by their parents.

    D. children would rather talk and read books than be on screens.

47. **Which conclusion is *not* supported by the article?**

    A. The author thinks kids are on their screens too much.

    B. The author thinks technology is negatively impacting children.

    C. The author thinks parents do not know how to discipline their children.

    D. The author thinks parents need to do more to help draw kids away from technology.

SECTION III. VOCABULARY & GENERAL KNOWLEDGE

You have 50 minutes to complete 50 questions.

1. Which of the following prefixes means "<u>large</u>"?

   A. con-   C. macro-

   B. rupt-   D. micro-

2. Select the meaning of the underlined word in the sentence.

   The senator had an <u>immutable</u> opposition to the bill and did everything she could to prevent it from passing.

   A. Fanatical   C. Dispassionate

   B. Questionable   D. Unchangeable

3. A <u>neophyte</u> is someone who

   A. works hard.

   B. knows a lot.

   C. is very curious.

   D. is new to something.

4. Which of the following root words means "<u>city</u>"?

   A. post   C. poly

   B. port   D. poli

5. Which of the following prefixes means <u>beneath</u>?

   A. inter-   C. port-

   B. trans-   D. infra-

6. Select the meaning of the underlined word in the sentence.

   He loves to use <u>hyperbole</u> in his writing to make his pieces more interesting.

   A. Details   C. Mystery

   B. Dialogue   D. Exaggeration

7. *Circumvent* means to

   A. find a way over.

   B. find a way under.

   C. find a way around.

   D. find a way through.

8. Which of the following suffixes means "<u>in the manner of</u>"?

   A. -ly   C. -less

   B. -ed   D. -ion

9. Which of the following root words means "<u>cut</u>"?

   A. cert   C. clar

   B. cise   D. cede

10. Which of the following prefixes means "<u>across</u>"?

    A. demi-   C. com-

    B. dia-   D. hypo-

11. The use of the suffix *-cide* in the word *genocide* indicates what?

    A. Many people have fallen ill.

    B. Many people have suffered.

    C. Many people have been killed.

    D. Many people have lost everything.

12. What is the best definition of the word *genuflect*?

    A. Sit   C. Stroll

    B. Bow   D. Stand

13. Which of the following root words means "<u>thankful</u>"?

    A. grat   C. gram

    B. gran   D. graph

14. What is the best definition of the word *transcontinental*?

   A. Near the continent

   B. Inside the continent

   C. Across the continent

   D. Outside the continent

15. Which of the following suffixes means "relating to" or "resembling"?

   A. -ular   C. -phile

   B. -ware   D. -wise

16. Which of the following root words means "life"?

   A. anti   C. anim

   B. arch   D. ambul

17. Which of the following prefixes means "short"?

   A. bio-   C. bene-

   B. bibl-   D. brev-

18. The use of the prefix *omni-* in the word *omnivore* indicates what about an animal?

   A. It eats only meat

   B. It eats only plants

   C. It eats both meat and plants

   D. It eats neither meat nor plants

19. Select the meaning of the underlined word in the sentence.

Susan is known as a business <u>magnate</u> and is at the top of her industry.

   A. A mischievous and evil person

   B. A wealthy and powerful person

   C. A giving and supportive person

   D. A knowledgeable and informed person

20. What is the best definition of the word *loquacious*?

   A. Selfish   C. Talkative

   B. Friendly   D. Resentful

21. Which of the following suffixes means "<u>a place for</u>"?

   A. -ation   C. -ative

   B. -arium   D. -arian

22. Select the context clue from the following sentence that helps you define the multiple meaning word <u>pupils</u>.

The doctor had to dilate the patient's pupils, so she could examine his eyes.

   A. "doctor"   C. "examine"

   B. "patient's" D. "eyes"

23. Select the meaning of the underlined word in the sentence based on the context clues.

The landscape of the tundra was <u>stark</u> and contained nothing but flat, open land.

   A. Vast   C. Bright

   B. Plain   D. Beautiful

24. Select the context clue from the following sentence that helps you define the word <u>ferocious</u>.

Cape buffaloes are very <u>ferocious</u> creatures; they are known to attack not only animals but moving vehicles.

   A. "creatures" C. "animals"

   B. "attack"   D. "moving"

25. Select the word from the following sentence that has more than one meaning.

    In the United States, the custom is to shake hands with someone when you meet them for the first time.

    A. Custom   C. First

    B. Meet   D. Time

26. Select the word from the following sentence that has more than one meaning.

    The caterer made a fruit punch for the party that was absolutely delicious.

    A. Caterer   C. Punch

    B. Fruit   D. Delicious

27. Select the correct definition of the underlined word that has multiple meanings in the sentence.

    Harriet has done a <u>fair</u> bit of coaching, so she was chosen to help out the girls' varsity basketball team.

    A. Honest   C. Attractive

    B. Cloudless   D. Reasonable

28. Select the context clue from the following sentence that helps you define the word <u>dreary</u>.

    The gray clouds made the day feel dreary.

    A. "gray"

    B. "clouds"

    C. "day"

    D. "feel"

29. Select the word from the following sentence that has more than one meaning.

    The committee met to discuss every angle of the problem they were trying to solve.

    A. Committee   C. Angle

    B. Discuss   D. Solve

30. Select the correct definition of the underlined word that has multiple meanings in the sentence.

    The bodybuilder has a powerful <u>trunk</u> since he lifts weights every day.

    A. The torso of a human body

    B. The main woody stem of a tree

    C. The elongated nose of an elephant

    D. A large storage box with a hinged lid

31. Select the context clue from the following sentence that helps you define the multiple meaning word <u>plate</u>.

    When Professor Higgins retired, he removed his name plate and kept it as a memento.

    A. "professor"

    B. "retired"

    C. "name"

    D. "memento"

32. Select the context clue from the following sentence that helps you define the word <u>erratic</u>.

    The skier became erratic after encountering some ice on the course.

    A. "skier"

    B. "encountering"

    C. "ice"

    D. "course"

33. Select the word from the following sentence that has more than one meaning.

After many hours of playing, Elliot finally won the chess match.

A. Hours

B. Playing

C. Chess

D. Match

34. Select the correct definition of the underlined word that has multiple meanings in the sentence.

Stella was pleased since her university offered a wide range of interesting courses.

A. An assortment of things

B. A large area of open land

C. A line or series of mountains

D. The scope of a person's knowledge

35. Select the context clue from the following sentence that helps you define the multiple meaning word mask.

Charlie tried to mask his habit of biting his nails by hiding when he did it.

A. "habit"

B. "biting"

C. "hiding"

D. "did"

36. Select the meaning of the underlined word in the sentence based on the context clues.

In the early fall the temperature tends to fluctuate a lot, so I never know what clothes to wear.

A. Vary

B. Rise

C. Fall

D. Stabilize

37. Select the context clue from the following sentence that helps you define the word insatiable.

The teenager has such an insatiable appetite that he eats frequently.

A. "teenager"

B. "appetite"

C. "eats "

D. "frequently"

38. Select the word from the following sentence that has more than one meaning.

After he failed his physics test, my brother began to channel his anger toward me.

A. Failed

B. Test

C. Channel

D. Anger

39. Select the correct definition of the underlined word that has more than one meaning in the sentence.

The nursing students were learning about the human figure with a life-sized dummy and other plastic models.

A. A shape or form

B. A person who is regarded in a special way

C. A diagram or picture

D. A value expressed in numbers

40. Which of the following is the term for the medical screening of patients to determine their priority?

A. Triage

B. Observation

C. Examination

D. Prescreening

41. Which of the following root words means "bones of the fingers and toes"?

A. Patell

B. Pector

C. Phalang

D. Pancreat

42. In this sentence, the suffix indicates that the doctor plans to do an excision on which body part?

The doctor needs to perform an appendectomy on the patient.

A. Abdomen   C. Appendage

B. Appendix   D. Adam's Apple

43. Based on your knowledge of medical roots, prefixes, and suffixes, which of the following words means "a disease of the intestines"?

A. Myopathy

B. Osteopathy

C. Enteropathy

D. Encephalopathy

44. Which of the following suffixes means "decay of"?

A. -osis   C. -sepsis

B. -stasis   D. -sclerosis

45. Based on your knowledge of roots, prefixes, and suffixes, what does *posterior* mean?

A. Toward the back   C. On the side

     D. At the top

B. Toward the front

46. Adding which of the following suffixes to *psycho* would describe the area of study focused on how medicine affects the brain?

A. -pathy

B. -ology

C. -logist

D. -pharmacology

47. Select the meaning of the underlined word in the sentence to complete the follow-up sentence.

The patient went to an <u>orthopedic</u> surgeon.

An orthopedic surgeon repairs anything that's part of the

A. nervous system.

B. reproductive system.

C. respiratory system.

D. musculoskeleton system.

48. Read the following sentence.

The doctor was treating the patient for thoracic pain.

What kind of pain was the patient experiencing?

A. Chest pain

B. Throat pain

C. Stomach pain

D. Lower back pain

49. Which root word means "reproduction"?

A. Gen   C. Gnos

B. Ger   D. Goni

50. Which of the following words means "pain of the kidneys"?

A. Nephralgia   C. Nephrotomy

B. Nephrology   D. Nephropathic

SECTION IV. GRAMMAR

You have 50 minutes to complete 50 questions.

1. **Which of the following spellings is correct?**

   A. Posibility

   B. Possibility

   C. Possibilitie

   D. Possibillity

2. **Which of the following spellings is correct?**

   A. Lonliness

   B. Lonelines

   C. Loneliness

   D. Loneleness

3. **Which of the following spellings is correct?**

   A. Prununciation

   B. Pronuncietion

   C. Pronunciation

   D. Pronounciation

4. **Which of the following spellings is correct?**

   A. Depindant

   B. Dependint

   C. Dependunt

   D. Dependent

5. **Which word(s) in the following sentence should NOT be capitalized?**

   The President Is Elected By The People.

   A. The, Is, By, and The

   B. Is, Elected, By, The

   C. Is, Elected, By, The, People

   D. President, Is, Elected, By, The, People

6. **Which word(s) in the following sentence should NOT be capitalized?**

   I Met Uncle John For Lunch Yesterday.

   A. Met, For, Lunch, and Yesterday

   B. Met, Uncle, John, For, and Lunch

   C. Met, John, For, Lunch, and Yesterday

   D. Met, Uncle, For, Lunch, and Yesterday

7. **Which word(s) in the following sentence should NOT be capitalized?**

   The Battle Of The Bulge Was The Last Major Battle Of World War II.

   A. Was, The, Last, Major, and Of

   B. Of, The, Was, The, Last, and Of

   C. Of, The, Was, The, Last, Major, Battle, and Of

   D. Battle, Of, The, Bulge, Was, The, Last, Major, Battle, Of, World, and War

8. **Which word(s) in the following sentence should NOT be capitalized?**

   The South Has Good Food.

   A. South and Has

   B. Has, Good, and Food

   C. South, Has, and Good

   D. South, Has, Good, and Food

9. **Which sentence is incorrect?**

   A. I hate you!

   B. When does the movie start?

   C. I go to bed early so I do not feel tired.

   D. You should drink eight glasses of water a day.

10. **Which of the following sentences is correct?**

    A. I asked Scott, How was your day?

    B. Scott said, it was awesome.

    C. He claimed, "My history presentation was great!"

    D. I said, That's wonderful!

11. **Which sentence is correct?**

    A. What is wrong.

    B. Honesty is the best policy.

    C. You dont need an umbrella.

    D. A band needs a guitarist singer and drummer.

12. **Which of the following sentences is correct?**

    A. Ashley cant ride a bike.

    B. Ashleys parents never taught her.

    C. Its an impossible task for her.

    D. Ashley's determined to learn.

13. **Which words in the following sentence are proper nouns?**

    Matthew had a meeting with his supervisor on Tuesday.

    A. Matthew, meeting

    B. Matthew, Tuesday

    C. meeting, supervisor

    D. supervisor, Tuesday

14. **Which words in the following sentence are common nouns?**

    The crowd cheered as Dr. King gave an inspiring speech.

    A. cheered, gave

    B. crowd, speech

    C. inspiring, speech

    D. crowd, Dr. King, speech

15. **Which word is a correct plural form?**

    A. Deer   C. Octopuses

    B. Babys   D. Brother-in-laws

16. **Which type of noun is the underlined word?**

    One thing I cannot tolerate is <u>dishonesty</u>.

    A. Plural noun   C. Abstract noun

    B. Proper noun   D. Concrete noun

17. **Which word in the following sentence is a pronoun?**

    The driver checked her side mirror.

    A. The   C. side

    B. her   D. driver

18. **Which word in the following sentence is a pronoun?**

    Maria washed Pavel's car for him.

    A. for   C. Maria

    B. him   D. Pavel's

19. **Which word is a subject pronoun?**

    A. He   C. Him

    B. Us   D. Our

20. Which word is an adverb that describes the underlined verb?

The man <u>spoke</u> to us wisely.

A. man
C. us

B. to
D. wisely

21. Which word in the following sentence is an adjective?

Washington, Jefferson, and Adams were founding fathers of the United States.

A. and
C. fathers

B. founding
D. of

22. Which word in the following sentence is an adverb?

We should go outside.

A. We
C. go

B. should
D. outside

23. Which word in the following sentence is an adjective?

The opera singer's voice, poise, and costume were all perfect.

A. voice
C. costume

B. poise
D. perfect

24. Which word is <u>not</u> a conjunction?

A. Or
C. So

B. The
D. But

25. What is the object of the underlined preposition?

I found our cat <u>under</u> the table by the window next to the TV.

A. our cat
C. the window

B. the table
D. the TV

26. Which word is <u>not</u> a preposition?

A. over
C. beside

B. without
D. what

27. Identify the prepositional phrase in the following sentence.

The show got great reviews, so we plan to see it on Saturday.

A. got great reviews
C. see it

B. so we plan
D. on Saturday

28. Why is the following <u>not</u> a correct sentence?

The clown sad.

A. It does not have a verb.

B. It does not have a noun.

C. The verb tense is incorrect.

D. The words are in the wrong order.

29. Which word <u>cannot</u> be used to complete the following sentence?

____ Stephanie and her brother take classes at the university?

A. Do
C. Can

B. Will
D. Are

30. Select the helping verb that correctly completes the following sentence.

After I ____ watched *The Godfather*, I immediately watched its two sequels.

A. did
C. had

B. was
D. have

31. Which part of the following sentence is the predicate?

Mai and her friend Oksana love to ride roller coasters.

A. Mai and her friend Oksana

B. and her friend Oksana

C. love to ride roller coasters

D. roller coasters

32. **What is the verb in the following sentence?**

   It's time for lunch.

   A. It
   B. is
   C. time
   D. lunch

33. **Which subject is third person singular?**

   A. I
   B. He
   C. We
   D. You

34. **Which part of the following sentence is the predicate?**

   My granddaughter was born on January 18.

   A. My granddaughter
   B. was
   C. was born on January 18
   D. January 18

35. **Which of the following options would complete the above sentence to make it a simple sentence?**

   You can see the wonders of our country

   _____

   A. on a road trip.
   B. take a road trip.
   C. and, on a road trip.
   D. rather than taking a road trip.

36. **Which of the following is an example of a simple sentence?**

   A. Although termites are insects.
   B. Termites are very industrious insects.
   C. Termites are insects, and they are very industrious.
   D. Because termites are insects, they are very industrious.

37. **Which of the following is an example of a simple sentence?**

   A. Calcium for bones.
   B. Calcium makes bones strong.
   C. Calcium is necessary it makes bones strong.
   D. Calcium is good for bones, so people need it.

38. **Which of the following is an example of a complex sentence?**

   A. Tabitha tried rock climbing, having a fear of heights.
   B. Tabitha tried rock climbing; fear of heights.
   C. Tabitha tried rock climbing having a fear of heights.
   D. Tabitha tried rock climbing having a fear of heights.

39. **Identify the independent clause in the following sentence.**

   You need to call your mother as soon as you get home.

   A. You need to call your mother
   B. As soon as you get home
   C. You get home
   D. You need to call

40. **Identify the type of clause.**

   She ate her lunch late.

   A. Dependent clause
   B. Subordinate clause
   C. Independent clause
   D. Coordinate clause

41. **Identify the type of clause.**

    When she went to the movie.

    A. Main clause

    B. Coordinate clause

    C. Independent clause

    D. Dependent or subordinate clause

42. **Identify the independent clause in the following sentence.**

    I began swimming every day, because it is healthy to exercise.

    A. I began swimming every day

    B. Because it is healthy to exercise

    C. It is healthy to exercise

    D. I began swimming

43. **Which word or phrase in the following sentence is not a modifier?**

    The woman found her lost earring yesterday.

    A. found   C. lost

    B. her   D. yesterday

44. **Which word or phrase in the following sentence is not a modifier?**

    Several tigers escaped from the zoo last night.

    A. Several   C. from the zoo

    B. escaped   D. last night

45. **Which word or phrase does the underlined modifier describe?**

    Despite their talent and hard work, the band had trouble selling records.

    A. the band   C. selling

    B. had trouble   D. records

46. **Which word or phrase is not a modifier?**

    Relieved that the grueling trial was over, the lawyer took a much-needed vacation.

    A. Relieved that the grueling trial was over

    B. grueling

    C. took

    D. much-needed

47. **Which of the following verbs cannot take a direct object?**

    A. Snore   C. Choose

    B. Watch   D. Bake

48. **Which verbs in the following sentence have indirect objects?**

    I told them my opinion when I said that giving their daughter a gerbil for her birthday was a bad idea.

    A. told, said   C. said, was

    B. told, giving   D. giving, was

49. **What part of speech correctly describes the underlined word in the following sentence?**

    I don't think you should give her that.

    A. Direct object   C. Verb

    B. Indirect object   D. Preposition

50. **What part of speech correctly describes the underlined phrase in the following sentence?**

    The mother fed the baby from a bottle.

    A. Subject

    B. Direct object

    C. Indirect object

    D. Object of the preposition

SECTION V. BIOLOGY

You have 25 minutes to complete 25 questions.

1. During protein synthesis in a cell, the primary structure of the protein consists of a linear chain of monomers. What is another way to describe this structure?

   A. A linear chain of fatty acids that are hydrogen-bonded together

   B. A linear chain of nucleotides that are hydrogen-bonded together

   C. A linear chain of amino acids that are covalently bonded together

   D. A linear chain of monosaccharides that are covalently bonded together

2. Which is a classification level in the Linnaean system?

   A. Achaea   C. Genus

   B. Domain   D. Ursidae

3. Which of the following helps differentiate a non-living thing from a living thing?

   A. Energy processing

   B. Behavior in nature

   C. Occurrence in nature

   D. Description of habitat

4. What standard is used to make comparisons in experiments?

   A. Sample size

   B. Control group

   C. Dependent variable

   D. Independent variable

5. _____ bonds are used to join water molecules together.

   A. Covalent   C. Ionic

   B. Hydrogen   D. Peptide

6. Which of the following is produced during the citric acid cycle?

   A. Electrons   C. Pyruvate

   B. NADH   D. Cellulose

7. Which is a characteristic of prokaryotes?

   A. They are classified as animal cells.

   B. These are known to be single-celled organisms.

   C. The cytoplasm contains a membrane-bound nucleus.

   D. Flagella and pili are attached to their outer cell surface.

8. A scientist discovers a cell that has a nucleus and is 15mm in size. What type of cell is this classified as?

   A. Eukaryote   C. Bacteria

   B. Achaea   D. Prokaryote

9. Which of the following is most likely absent in prokaryotic cells?

   A. Cilia   C. Lysosomes

   B. Flagella   D. Ribosomes

10. In a cell, the mitochondrion is to supplying energy as a Golgi apparatus is to _____.

    A. housing DNA

    B. storing water

    C. digesting food

    D. packaging proteins

11. Which organelle is separated from the cytoplasm due to the presence of its own membrane?

A. Mitochondrion

B. Nucleus

C. Ribosome

D. Vacuole

12. What raw inorganic material would an autotroph most likely use to create chemical energy for growth?

A. carbon dioxide

B. minerals in soil

C. decaying matter

D. sugar molecules

13. Which of the following characteristics is unique to all prokaryotes?

A. Creates gametes

B. Requires meiosis

C. Uses photosynthesis

D. Reproduces asexually

14. Which process is part of photosynthesis?

A. Anaphase

B. Glycolysis

C. Calvin cycle

D. Pyruvate oxidation

15. Which organism could survive without cellular respiration?

A. Cyanobacteria   C. Plant

B. Human   D. Racoon

16. Which organism most likely produces offspring asexually?

A. Bacteria   C. Humans

B. Birds   D. Lions

17. DNA _____ during the synthesis phase in mitosis.

A. splits in half

B. triples in size

C. doubles in size

D. breaks into small pieces

18. Sister chromatids and centromeres are found in a _____ chromosome.

A. replicated

B. duplicated

C. histone absent

D. loosely condensed

19. Which of the following is the base that will bind with cytosine?

A. Adenine   C. Guanine

B. Cytosine   D. Thymine

20. According to Mendel's observations, which of the following is a theory of heredity?

A. Individuals receive one allele from each parent

B. Genotype determines the physical appearance of a person.

C. Parents transmit genetic traits directly to offspring without genes.

D. All phenotypic traits come from either the mom or dad, but not both.

21. Several descendants in a family tree are known to have green eyes and brown curly hair. These characteristics are also known as _____ .

A. alleles   C. genotypes

B. genes   D. phenotypes

22. Samantha uses a Punnett Square to estimate what a litter of puppies will look like. She crosses homozygous dominant trait of brown fur with a homozygous recessive trait for curly fur. Which of the following most likely designates the dominant trait in this Punnett Square?

    A. F   C. ff

    B. FF   D. f

23. Which of the following is a component of a chromosome?

    A. Centromere   C. Homologue

    B. Gamete   D. Ribose

24. What is DNA packaged in?

    A. Chromosomes   C. Centromeres

    B. Nucleotides   D. Phosphate

25. Adenine is a nucleotide base that pairs with _____.

    A. guanine   C. uracil

    B. cytosine   D. thymine

SECTION VI. CHEMISTRY

You have 25 minutes to complete 25 questions.

1. **What is a treatment group?**

   A. A type of placebo

   B. A baseline measure

   C. The outcome of interest

   D. The variable being manipulated

2. **Three different dispersants that are used to break up oil in water are evaluated for their effectiveness. Dispersant A has a concentration of 10m, dispersant B has a concentration of 7m, and dispersant C has a concentration of 3m. Each dispersant is separately poured into a solution of water and oil. The amount of time it takes each dispersant to disperse the oil is recorded. Which of the following statements describes the positive correlation observed in this study?**

   A. Oil remains suspended in solution despite dispersant addition.

   B. As more dispersant is added to the water, more oil is dispersed.

   C. Dispersant C is the least effective at dispersing oil in the solution of water.

   D. When a high concentration of dispersant is added, less oil disperses in water.

3. **Time is measured using a**

   A. barometer.

   B. stopwatch.

   C. graduated cylinder.

   D. triple beam balance.

4. **Empirical evidence is**

   A. repeatable by multiple scientists.

   B. used to explain the placebo effect.

   C. created using deductive reasoning.

   D. data that contains metric base units.

5. **Which of the following atoms will have an overall negative charge?**

   A. 9 protons, 10 neutrons, 9 electrons

   B. 12 protons, 13 neutrons, 10 electrons

   C. 14 protons, 14 neutrons, 10 electrons

   D. 15 protons, 16 neutrons, 18 electrons

6. **In the periodic table, which element is in period 5 and group 4?**

   A. Manganese   C. Vanadium

   B. Molybdenum   D. Zirconium

7. **What is the charge of the nucleus of an atom?**

   A. Neutral

   B. Positive

   C. Negative

   D. Not enough information

8. **Which of the following atoms will have an overall positive charge?**

   A. 9 protons, 10 neutrons, 10 electrons

   B. 10 protons, 10 neutrons, 10 electrons

   C. 11 protons, 12 neutrons, 10 electrons

   D. 14 protons, 14 neutrons, 18 electrons

9. **How many ounces are in 3 cups?**

   A. 5   C. 11

   B. 8   D. 24

10. It is advantageous to use the English system when

   A. converting units using multiples of 10.

   B. describing a reported value using tons.

   C. working with functionally related base units.

   D. communicating information around the world.

11. How many feet are in a mile?

   A. 3   C. 2,000

   B. 12   D. 5,280

12. How many grams are equivalent to a 25.0 ounce container?

   A. 0.883   C. 226

   B. 53.3   D. 707

13. In which of the following phases are particles of a substance generally closest together?

   A. Gas   C. Plasma

   B. Liquid   D. Solid

14. During which of the following phase changes will the cohesion between the particles in a substance increase?

   A. Solid to gas   C. Gas to liquid

   B. Liquid to gas   D. Solid to liquid

15. Compare the melting points of three metals: gold (1063°C), lead (328°C), and mercury (-38.9°C). Which of the following statements is true regarding intermolecular forces of these metals?

   A. The intermolecular forces are strongest between atoms of gold.

   B. The intermolecular forces are strongest between atoms of mercury.

   C. The intermolecular forces of these metals are stronger after they melt.

   D. The intermolecular forces of these metals get stronger as they are heated.

16. What is polar molecule?

   A. A molecule that contains oxygen

   B. A molecule that is repulsed by water

   C. A molecule that is attracted to water

   D. A molecule that has slight charges on each end

17. Why does oxygen diffuse out of lungs into the bloodstream?

   A. The oxygen is repulsed by the blood.

   B. The oxygen is being pulled into the blood.

   C. The oxygen is polar, and the blood has the opposite charge.

   D. The oxygen is going from a higher area of concentration to a lower one.

18. How do zinc and sulfur react to form a compound?

   A. Zinc and sulfur will share electrons.

   B. Sulfur will transfer electrons to zinc.

   C. Zinc will transfer electrons to sulfur.

   D. Zinc and sulfur do not react with each other.

19. The first and second energy levels of a neutral atom are full, and the third energy level contains three electrons. To which group does this element belong?

A. Group 3   C. Group 10

B. Group 8   D. Group 13

20. Which of the following statements is true regarding bond that forms between two oxygen atoms in a molecule of O_2?

A. The oxygen atoms share electrons equally.

B. One oxygen atom pulls harder on shared electrons than the other.

C. One atom of oxygen loses two electrons, while the other gains two electrons.

D. There is not enough information to describe the bond in a molecule of oxygen.

21. What is the maximum amount of $KClO_3$ that can be dissolved in 50 grams of water at 30°C?

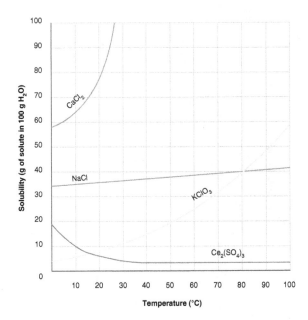

A. 5 grams   C. 20 grams

B. 10 grams   D. 70 grams

22. What is the maximum amount of NaCl that will dissolve in 100 grams of water at 90°C?

Solubility Curves

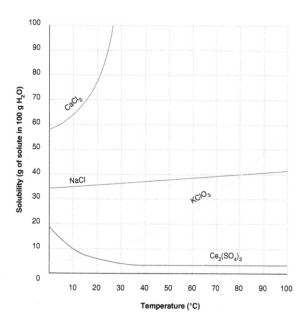

A. 34 grams   C. 40 grams

B. 38 grams   D. 47 grams

23. A Lewis acid is a substance that

A. accepts hydrogen ions.

B. ionizes completely in solution.

C. partially dissociates in solution.

D. donates a lone pair of electrons.

24. A researcher identifies an unknown solution to have a pH of 3. What characteristic does the researcher most likely write down about this solution?

A. Sour in taste

B. Weak electrolyte

C. Minimally corrosive

D. Slippery to the touch

25. Which product completes the following acid-base reaction?

$$H_2SO_4 + 2KOH \longrightarrow ?$$

A. H_3O^+ C. K_2SO_4

B. HSO_3^- D. $KHSO_4$

Section VII. Anatomy & Physiology

You have 25 minutes to complete 25 questions.

1. When dissecting an organ, sometimes a _____ cut needs to be made to divide the organ into top and bottom halves.

   A. coronal
   B. midsagittal
   C. sagittal
   D. transverse

2. The ventral cavity (front of the body) contains _____ major cavities.

   A. two
   B. three
   C. five
   D. nine

3. What is the purpose of the superior vena cava?

   A. Flow blood into the pulmonary artery
   B. Facilitate blood drainage into the right ventricle
   C. Carries deoxygenated blood from the upper half of the body to the right atrium
   D. Saturate the body tissues with a large volume of blood

4. What happens after blood coagulation?

   A. Platelet plug forms.
   B. Fibrin mesh is created.
   C. Blood vessels contract.
   D. Wounded site is closed.

5. Which body system works with the respiratory system to aid in blood pH regulation?

   A. Digestive
   B. Integumentary
   C. Nervous
   D. Urinary

6. As air rushes out of the lungs, the

   A. rib cage shortens.
   B. bronchioles shrink.
   C. diaphragm relaxes.
   D. lungs change shape.

7. One of the symptoms of hepatitis that makes it dangerous is that it

   A. alters the blood content of the area.
   B. replaces dead liver cells with scar tissue.
   C. covers the damaged liver cells with adipose tissue.
   D. converts the area of dead liver cells into non-porous tissue.

8. Where are the sublingual salivary glands located?

   A. Near the ears
   B. Below the jaw
   C. Under the tongue
   D. Beside the sinuses

9. The ova are analogous to which component of the male reproductive system?

   A. Foreskin
   B. Scrotum
   C. Sperm
   D. Testis

10. The male reproductive system includes _____.

    A. the penis and epididymis
    B. the vas deferens and uterus
    C. the penis and Fallopian tube
    D. the penis, scrotum, and cervix

171

11. In which of the following segments do both secretion and reabsorption occur?

    A. Loop of Henle

    B. Collecting duct

    C. Bowman's capsule

    D. Distal convoluted tubule

12. Which activity is most likely associated with microscopic urinalysis?

    A. Observing the color of urine

    B. Determining red blood cell count

    C. Identifying the presence of creatinine

    D. Noting the turbidity of a urine sample

13. What body system is the skeletal system most closely associated with when hematopoiesis happens?

    A. Urinary system

    B. Digestive system

    C. Muscular system

    D. Cardiovascular system

14. What bone type is the patella classified as?

    A. Flat bone   C. Short bone

    B. Long bone   D. Sesamoid bone

15. The cytoplasm of the skeletal muscle fiber is referred to as the _____.

    A. myofibril   C. sarcolemma

    B. perimysium   D. sarcoplasm

16. What happens after myosin heads attach to thin actin myofilaments?

    A. Crossbridges are formed.

    B. Molecules of ATP are released.

    C. The myosin head is reenergized.

    D. Calcium ion concentration increases.

17. Which contributes to the striated appearance of skeletal muscle?

    A. Presence of myosin filaments

    B. Cylindrical shape of the muscle

    C. Change in length of the sarcomere

    D. Quantity of myofibrils in a muscle fiber

18. Which describes the primary function of hair?

    A. Protect the surface of the skin

    B. Prevent heat loss from the head

    C. Fight off various microbial infections

    D. Excrete toxic substances from the body

19. The hair bulb contains actively growing _____ cells.

    A. basal   C. epithelial

    B. epidermal   D. merkel

20. The hypothalamus works directly with the _____ to control the body using hormones.

    A. amygdala   C. pituitary gland

    B. hippocampus   D. skeletal muscle

21. Which neuroglia produces myelin sheaths?

    A. Satellite cells

    B. Schwann cells

    C. Microglial cells

    D. Ependymal cells

22. Some intercellular chemical signals diffuse across cell membranes and bind to intracellular receptors. What are the two factors that enable this to occur?

    A. They are small and soluble.

    B. They are large and soluble.

    C. They are small and insoluble.

    D. They are large and insoluble.

23. Which of the following hormones would cause skin color to become darker?

    A. Follicle-stimulating

    B. Growth-stimulating

    C. Thyroid-stimulating

    D. Melanocyte-stimulating

24. Once the third line of defense has begun, which of the following has already occurred?

    A. The B cells flagged the pathogen.

    B. Histamines blocked the pathogen.

    C. The patrolling macrophages missed the pathogen.

    D. Killer T cells were unable to destroy the pathogen.

25. Allergies are a result of_____.

    A. histamines building up in the sinuses

    B. the immune system reacting to pollen

    C. the immune system doing too good a job

    D. the body's immune system breaking down

Section VIII. Physics

You have 50 minutes to complete 25 questions.

1. If a plane has a velocity that changes but is always in the same direction, which statement about its speed is true?

   A. The plane's speed is 0.

   B. The plane's speed is varying.

   C. The plane's speed is negative.

   D. The plane's speed is constant.

2. What is the acceleration of a 9.7-kilogram object moving at a velocity (2.3, 8.9) meters per second and subject to a net force of (3.2, –1.8) newtons?

   A. (–0.093, 1.1) m/s²

   B. (0.24, 0.92) m/s²

   C. (0.33, –0.19) m/s²

   D. (0.56, 0.73) m/s²

3. A child throws a ball directly upward from the ground with an initial speed of 45 meters per second. How long will the ball take to return to the ground?

   A. 1.4 seconds

   B. 2.0 seconds

   C. 3.0 seconds

   D. 9.2 seconds

4. Given vector $\vec{u}$ = (–4, 6) and scalar a = 3, what is $a\vec{u}$?

   A. (–12, 6)

   B. (–12, 18)

   C. (–1, 6)

   D. (–1, 9)

5. A cannonball is fired with an initial vertical velocity of 130 meters per second and an initial horizontal velocity of 450 meters per second. If it hits the ground 12 seconds after it is fired, how far did it travel?

   A. 1,600 meters

   B. 3,800 meters

   C. 5,400 meters

   D. 7,000 meters

6. The friction force in newtons on a certain type of sliding block is 0.050 times the block's mass in kilograms. What is the minimum horizontal force that must be applied to slide a 230-kilogram block?

   A. 2.2×10^{-4} N

   B. 12 N

   C. 230 N

   D. 4,600 N

7. A car is moving east at 20 meters per second. In what direction is the force of friction?

   A. East

   B. North

   C. South

   D. West

8. An object has a constant nonzero speed but a randomly varying velocity. Which term best describes its motion?

   A. Linear

   B. Nonlinear

   C. Rotational

   D. Stationary

9. A satellite is 6.7×10^6 meters from the center of Earth. If it maintains a circular orbit, what is its speed? (The acceleration due to gravity is 9.8 m/s².)

   A. 8.3×10^2 m/s

   B. 8.1×10^3 m/s

   C. 6.8×10^5 m/s

   D. 6.6×10^7 m/s

10. Which set of information about an object in uniform circular motion is sufficient to determine the object's velocity?

   A. Frequency, mass, period

   B. Centrifugal force, mass, radius of motion

   C. Angular frequency, centripetal force, period

   D. Angular frequency, centripetal acceleration, mass

11. What kind of force exists between an electron and a proton?

   A. No net force

   B. A repulsive force

   C. A rotational force

   D. An attractive force

12. An oceanographer has set a post in the water near shore to study waves before a hurricane. If she finds that the waves are 75 feet apart and a trough arrives every 25 seconds, what is the frequency?

   A. 0.013 Hz   C. 25 Hz

   B. 0.040 Hz   D. 75 Hz

13. A ray traveling in air strikes water at an angle of 30.0° from the normal. What will its angle be in the water? (Assume air has a refractive index of 1.00 and water has a refractive index of 1.30.)

   A. 22.6°   C. 39.0°

   B. 23.1°   D. 40.5°

14. Successive troughs of a sound wave arrive through a certain liquid every 0.040 seconds. If they are 100 feet apart, how fast are they traveling?

   A. 0.00040 feet per second

   B. 4.0 feet per second

   C. 25 feet per second

   D. 2,500 feet per second

15. Light traveling in a clear material of refractive index 2.1 enters air (refractive index 1.0) after hitting the interface between the two at a 15° angle. Which statement describes what the light will do?

   A. The light will experience no refraction.

   B. The light will reflect without any refraction.

   C. The light will refract toward the normal to the interface.

   D. The light will refract away from the normal to the interface.

16. A roller coaster car loaded with riders has a mass of 1490 kg. The car reaches its top speed of 26.8 m/s at the bottom of the first hill (along ground level). What was the height of the previous hill?

   A. 2.73 m   C. 36.6 m

   B. 19.2 m   D. 73.4 m

17. What two factors determine an object's kinetic energy?

   A. Mass and velocity

   B. Mass and acceleration

   C. Velocity and acceleration

   D. Distance and acceleration

18. What is the velocity of a 70 kg runner with a momentum of 700 $\frac{kg \cdot m}{s}$?

A. 5 $\frac{m}{s}$

B. 7 $\frac{m}{s}$

C. 10 $\frac{m}{s}$

D. 12 $\frac{m}{s}$

19. A track and field athlete holds a shot put of mass 7.3 kg at chin level 1.5 m above the ground. How much potential energy does the shot have? (Use g = 9.8 $\frac{m}{s^2}$)

A. 55 J

B. 110 J

C. 180 J

D. 230 J

20. At what separation distance do the 2,031,000 kg space shuttle and the 11,110 kg Hubble Space Telescope experience a 10.0 N force of gravitational attraction?

A. 0.156 m

B. 0.388 m

C. 1.56×10^{10} m

D. 3.88×10^{10} m

21. Which of the following best describes an electric current?

A. The storage of electric charge

B. The movement of electric charge

C. The energy required to move electric charge

D. The impedance of electric charge's movement

22. If an engineer converts magnetic fields into an electric potential difference, what is he employing?

A. Ohm's law

B. Electric flux

C. Coulomb's law

D. Electromagnetic induction

23. The magnetic flux near the end of a magnet is much greater than the magnetic flux farther away from the end. If the magnet moves away from a wire loop, what will happen?

A. The loop will rotate.

B. Nothing will happen.

C. A current will flow in the loop.

D. The loop will exert an electric force on the magnet.

24. An object carrying 5.00 coulombs of charge exerts 12,500 newtons of force on an object carrying 10.0 coulombs. How far apart are the objects? (Assume the electric constant is 9×10^9 when using units of newtons, coulombs, and meters.)

A. 1.00×10^2 meters

B. 2.50×10^3 meters

C. 6.00×10^3 meters

D. 3.60×10^9 meters

25. A 100-watt light bulb runs off a 120-volt source. If 0.83 amps flow through the bulb, what is its resistance?

A. 100 ohms

B. 120 ohms

C. 140 ohms

D. 270 ohms

HESI Practice Exam 3
Answer Key with Explanatory Answers

Section I. Mathematics

1. B. The correct solution is 30. Use the addition algorithm or a number line. Mental addition is also an option because the numbers are small. **Skill: Basic Addition and Subtraction.**

2. C. The correct solution is zero. Try a few examples: 6 – 6, 100 – 100, (–5) – (–5). All are equal to zero. **Skill: Basic Addition and Subtraction.**

3. D. The correct solution is not enough information. If you try a few examples, you will find that if the first number is less than the second, the difference is negative, but if the first number is greater than the second, the difference is positive. If the numbers are equal, the difference is 0. The question therefore provides too little information to choose A, B, or C. **Skill: Basic Addition and Subtraction.**

4. B. The correct solution is 77. The first step is to convert this problem to a math expression. The goal is to find the difference between how many minutes Kevin has for the exam and how many he has left after 43 minutes have elapsed. The expression would be 120 – 43. Carefully follow the subtraction algorithm (See below). The process will involve borrowing a digit twice.

$$\begin{array}{r} 120 \\ -\ 43 \\ \hline \end{array} \rightarrow \begin{array}{r} {\scriptstyle 110} \\ 1\overset{}{2}0 \\ -\ 43 \\ \hline 7 \end{array} \rightarrow \begin{array}{r} {\scriptstyle 0\ 1110} \\ \not{1}\not{2}0 \\ -\ 43 \\ \hline 77 \end{array}$$

Skill: Basic Addition and Subtraction.

5. B. The correct solution is 252. Carefully follow the addition algorithm (See below). The process involves carrying a digit twice.

$$\begin{array}{r} 154 \\ +\ 98 \\ \hline \end{array} \rightarrow \begin{array}{r} {\scriptstyle 1} \\ 154 \\ +\ 98 \\ \hline 2 \end{array} \rightarrow \begin{array}{r} {\scriptstyle 11} \\ 154 \\ +\ 98 \\ \hline 52 \end{array} \rightarrow \begin{array}{r} {\scriptstyle 11} \\ 154 \\ +\ 98 \\ \hline 252 \end{array}$$

Skill: Basic Addition and Subtraction.

6. B. Use the division algorithm. Because 127 is greater than 7 and 76, the process begins with all three digits in the dividend. **Skill: Basic Multiplication and Division.**

7. B. This expression only involves addition and subtraction, but its evaluation must go from left to right. **Skill: Basic Multiplication and Division.**

$$3 + 1 - 5 + 2 - 6$$
$$4 - 5 + 2 - 6$$
$$(-1) + 2 - 6$$
$$1 - 6$$
$$-5$$

8. C. Use the division algorithm. Determining the first digit of the quotient requires using the first three digits in the dividend. **Skill: Basic Multiplication and Division.**

9. B. When evaluating expressions with pvarentheses, begin with the innermost ones and work outward, following the order of operations. This case only involves addition and subtraction.

$$6 + (1 - (2 + (5 - (3 - 1))))$$
$$6 + (1 - (2 + (5 - 2)))$$
$$6 + (1 - (2 + 3))$$
$$6 + (1 - 5)$$
$$6 + (-4)$$
$$2$$

Skill: Basic Multiplication and Division.

10. C. Remember that division is the inverse of multiplication, so division and multiplication are related. Consider any example of division: multiplying the divisor and the quotient always yields the dividend. For example, $18 \div 6 = 3$ and $3 \times 6 = 18$. **Skill: Basic Multiplication and Division.**

11. C. The correct solution is 2.002 because 2.002 contains the smallest values in the tenths and hundredths places. **Skill: Decimals and Fractions.**

12. D. The correct solution is $\frac{2}{3}$ because $\frac{2}{3}$ has the smallest numerator when comparing to the other fractions with the same denominator. The fractions with a common denominator of 24 are

$$\frac{5}{6} = \frac{20}{24}, \frac{3}{4} = \frac{18}{24}, \frac{17}{24} = \frac{17}{24}, \frac{2}{3} = \frac{16}{24}.$$

Skill: Decimals and Fractions.

13. D. The correct answer is $2\frac{9}{10}$ because 290% as a fraction is $2\frac{90}{100} = 2\frac{9}{10}$. **Skill: Decimal and Fractions**

14. C. The correct solution is $\frac{1}{2}$ because $\frac{1}{2}$ has the largest numerator when comparing to the other fractions with the same denominator. The fractions with a common denominator of 20 are

$$\frac{3}{10} = \frac{6}{20}, \frac{2}{5} = \frac{8}{20}, \frac{1}{2} = \frac{10}{20}, \frac{1}{4} = \frac{5}{20}.$$

Skill: Decimals and Fractions.

15. B. The correct solution is 2 because $\frac{16}{5} \times \frac{5}{8} = \frac{80}{40} = 2$. **Skill: Multiplication and Division of Fractions.**

16. C. The correct solution is $1\frac{1}{2}$ because $\frac{2}{1} \times \frac{3}{4} = \frac{6}{4} = 1\frac{2}{4} = 1\frac{1}{2}$. **Skill: Multiplication and Division of Fractions.**

17. C. 36 is the correct answer because $\frac{8}{1} \times \frac{9}{2} = \frac{72}{2} = 36$. **Skill: Multiplication and Division of Fractions.**

18. B. The correct solution is $1\frac{1}{5}$ because $\frac{2}{5} \times \frac{3}{1} = \frac{6}{5} = 1\frac{1}{5}$. **Skill: Multiplication and Division of Fractions.**

19. C. The ratio is 23:35. The first part of the ratio is the number of people in group Y, which is 230. The second part is the number of people in either group, which is the sum $120 + 230 = 350$. The ratio is therefore 230:350 = 23:35. **Skill: Ratios, Proportions, and Percentages.**

20. A. The ratio is 4:11. A ratio is like a fraction of two numbers, although in this case the answer uses colon notation. The ratio of brand B to brand A is the number of brand-B cars divided by the number of brand-A cars. Reduce to lowest terms:

$$\frac{48}{132} = \frac{4}{11}$$

Skill: Ratios, Proportions, and Percentages.

21. D. The expression 0.04 is different from the others. The expression in answer A is a fraction, and it is equal to the ratio in answer B. Dividing 2 by 5 yields 0.4, which is equal to 40%. The option left is 0.04, which is different from the others. **Skill: Ratios, Proportions, and Percentages.**

22. A. As a ratio, 36% is 9:25. The most direct route is to convert 36% to a fraction, $\frac{36}{100}$, then reduce to lowest terms: $\frac{9}{25}$. The equivalent ratio in colon notation is 9:25. **Skill: Ratios, Proportions, and Percentages.**

23. B. The population's rate of increase was −6%. The solution in this case involves two steps. First, calculate the population's annual rate of change using the formula. It will yield the change in the number of individuals.

$$\frac{2{,}115 - 2{,}250}{1 \text{ year} - 0 \text{ year}} = -135 \text{ per year}$$

Second, divide the result by the initial population. Finally, convert to a percent.

$$\frac{-135 \text{ per year}}{2{,}250} = -0.06 \text{ per year}$$

$$(-0.06 \text{ per year}) \times 100\% = -6\% \text{ per year}$$

Since the question asks for the *annual* rate of increase, the "per year" can be dropped. Also, note that the answer must be negative to represent the decreasing population. **Skill: Ratios, Proportions, and Percentages.**

24. B. The correct solution is 0.099 kilometers. $99 \text{ m} \times \frac{1 \text{ km}}{1,000 \text{ m}} = \frac{99}{1,000} = 0.099$ km. **Skill: Standards of Measure.**

25. D. The correct solution is 1500. Add 1200 to the time, $1200 + 300 = 1500$. **Skill: Standards of Measure.**

26. B. The correct solution is 7:20 p.m. Subtract 1200 from the time, $1920 - 1200 = 7\!:\!20$ p.m. **Skill: Standards of Measure.**

27. D. The correct solution is 320 fluid ounces. $10 \text{ qt} \times \frac{2 \text{ pt}}{1 \text{ qt}} \times \frac{16 \text{ fl oz}}{1 \text{ pt}} = 320$ fl. oz. **Skill: Standards of Measure.**

28. A. The correct solution is 438.8 meters. $4{,}388 \text{ dm} \times \frac{1 \text{ m}}{10 \text{ dm}} = \frac{4{,}388}{10} = 438.8$ m. **Skill: Standards of Measure.**

29. C. The correct solution is 6.

$\frac{x}{2} = 3$	Subtract 5 from both sides of the equation.
$x = 6$	Multiply both sides of the equation by 2.

Skill: Equations with One Variable.

30. C. The correct solution is $x < -\frac{3}{5}$.

$3-x+4x+4 < 2(2-x)$	Multiply all terms by the least common denominator of 4 to eliminate the fractions.
$3-x+4x+4 < 4-2x$	Apply the distributive property.
$3x+7 < 4-2x$	Combine like terms on the left side of the inequality.
$5x+7 < 4$	Add $2x$ to both sides of the inequality.
$5x < -3$	Subtract 7 from both sides of the inequality.
$x < -\frac{3}{5}$	Divide both sides of the inequality by 5.

Skill: Equations with One Variable.

31. C. The correct solution is $\frac{4}{3}$.

$3x = 4$	Subtract 8 from both sides of the equation.
$x = \frac{4}{3}$	Divide both sides of the equation by 3.

Skill: Equations with One Variable.

32. A. The correct solution is $x > 2$.

$3x + 5 - 2x - 6 > 4 - 4x + 5$	Apply the distributive property.
$x - 1 > -4x + 9$	Combine like terms on both sides of the inequality.
$5x - 1 > 9$	Add $4x$ to both sides of the inequality.
$5x > 10$	Add 1 to both sides of the inequality.
$x > 2$	Divide both sides of the inequality by 5.

Skill: Equations with One Variable.

33. D. The correct solution is (-4, -8).

	The second equation is already solved for y.
$2(-x - 12) + x = -20$	Substitute $-x - 12$ in for y in the first equation.
$-2x - 24 + x = -20$	Apply the distributive property.
$-x - 24 = -20$	Combine like terms on the left side of the equation.
$-x = 4$	Add 24 to both sides of the equation.
$x = -4$	Divide both sides of the equation by -1.
$y = -(-4) - 12$	Substitute -4 in the second equation for x.
$y = 4 - 12 = -8$	Simplify using order of operations.

Skill: Equations with Two Variables.

34. D. The correct solutions are (2, -2) and (-2, 2).

$x^2 + (-x)^2 = 8$	Substitute $-x$ in for y in the second equation.
$x^2 + x^2 = 8$	Apply the exponent.
$2x^2 = 8$	Combine like terms on the left side of the equation.
$x^2 = 4$	Divide both sides of the equation by 2.
$x = \pm 2$	Apply the square root to both sides of the equation.
$y = -2$	Substitute 2 in the first equation.
$y = -(-2) = 2$	Substitute -2 in the first equation and multiply.

Skill: Equations with Two Variables.

35. A. The correct solution is (-2, 7).

	The first equation is already solved for y.
$-2x + 3 + x = 5$	Substitute $-2x + 3$ in for y in the second equation.
$-x + 3 = 5$	Combine like terms on the left side of the equation.
$-x = 2$	Subtract 3 from both sides of the equation.
$x = -2$	Divide both sides of the equation by -1.
$y = -2(-2) + 3$	Substitute -2 in the first equation for x.
$y = 4 + 3 = 7$	Simplify using order of operations.

Skill: Equations with Two Variables.

36. D. The correct graph has the two lines intersect at (-1, 2). **Skill: Equations with Two Variables.**

37. D. The correct graph has the two lines intersect at (5, 2). **Skill: Equations with Two Variables.**

38. C. The correct solution is $9\frac{3}{5}$ because $2\frac{2}{5} \times 4 = \frac{12}{5} \times \frac{4}{1} = \frac{48}{5} = 9\frac{3}{5}$ pounds of apples. **Skill: Solving Real World Mathematical Problems.**

39. B. The correct solution is -5 because $14(2) + 11(-3) = 28 + (-33) = -5$ points. **Skill: Solving Real World Mathematical Problems.**

40. B. The correct solution is $-\$85$ because $250 - (70 + 85 + 60 + 100 + 20) = 250 - 335 = -\$85$. **Skill: Solving Real World Mathematical Problems.**

41. B. The correct solution is 30 because $4(3) \div \frac{2}{5} = 12 \div \frac{2}{5} = \frac{12}{1} \times \frac{5}{2} = \frac{60}{2} = 30$ cups of water. **Skill: Solving Real World Mathematical Problems.**

42. A. The correct solution is 12 because the first company has about 600,000,000 orders and the second company has about 50,000,000 orders. So, the first company is about 12 times larger. **Skill: Powers, Exponents, Roots, and Radicals.**

43. C. The correct solution is y^4 because $\left(\frac{x^0}{y^{-2}}\right)^2 = \frac{x^{0 \times 2}}{y^{-2 \times 2}} = \frac{x^0}{y^{-4}} = \frac{1}{y^{-4}} = y^4$. **Skill: Powers, Exponents, Roots, and Radicals.**

44. C. The correct solution is 500 because 1×10^{-6} is 0.000001 and 2×10^{-9} is about 0.000000002. So, the lysosome is 500 times longer. **Skill: Powers, Exponents, Roots, and Radicals.**

45. B. The correct solution is $\frac{x^{20}}{625}$ because $\left(\frac{x^5}{5}\right)^4 = \frac{x^{5 \times 4}}{5^4} = \frac{x^{20}}{625}$. **Skill: Powers, Exponents, Roots, and Radicals.**

46. D. The correct solution is $-13, 13$ because the square root of 169 is 13. The values of -13 and 13 make the equation true. **Skill: Powers, Exponents, Roots, and Radicals.**

47. C. The correct solution is $12x^2 + 7x - 10$.

$$(4x + 5)(3x - 2) = 4x(3x - 2) + 5(3x - 2) = 12x^2 - 8x + 15x - 10 = 12x^2 + 7x - 10$$

Skill: Polynomials.

48. B. The correct solution is $(3x - 2)(9x^2 + 6x + 4)$. The expression $27x^3 - 8$ is rewritten as $(3x - 2)(9x^2 + 6x + 4)$ because the value of a is $3x$ and the value of b is 2. **Skill: Polynomials.**

49. A. The correct solution is $3x^3 - 6x^2 + 8x + 1$.

$$(-2x^2 + 8x) + (3x^3 - 4x^2 + 1) = 3x^3 + (-2x^2 - 4x^2) + 8x + 1 = 3x^3 - 6x^2 + 8x + 1$$

Skill: Polynomials.

50. C. The correct solution is $(4x + 11)(4x - 11)$. The expression $16x^2 - 121$ is rewritten as $(4x + 11)(4x - 11)$ because the value of a is $4x$ and the value of b is 11. **Skill: Polynomials.**

Section II. Reading Comprehension

1. D. The topic of this paragraph the benefits of dark chocolate. **Skill: Main Ideas, Topic Sentences, and Supporting Details.**

2. B. The second sentence of this paragraph leads the reader toward the main idea, which is that dark chocolate has health benefits. **Skill: Main Ideas, Topic Sentences, and Supporting Details.**

3. D. A popular recipe using dark chocolate as its main ingredient would be an off-topic sentence since it is not related to the main idea of the health benefits of dark chocolate. **Skill: Main Ideas, Topic Sentences, and Supporting Details.**

4. C. The description of the paragraph is not valid because the author of the paragraph ends with a warning to readers about its high caloric content. **Skill: Main Ideas, Topic Sentences, and Supporting Details.**

5. A. This statistic would be off-topic information in this paragraph because it is about all chocolate not the health benefits of dark chocolate. **Skill: Main Ideas, Topic Sentences, and Supporting Details.**

6. B. The main idea of the sentence is how kindergarten has changed. **Skill: Main Ideas, Topic Sentences, and Supporting Details.**

7. A. The sentence above conveys information about today's kindergartens being more like first grade classrooms from thirty years ago. This makes it most likely to fit into a persuasive paragraph about kindergarten not being developmentally appropriate for children. **Skill: Main Ideas, Topic Sentences, and Supporting Details.**

8. C. If the above sentence were a topic sentence, its supporting details would likely share information to develop the idea that kindergarten today looks very different from kindergarten years ago. **Skill: Main Ideas, Topic Sentences, and Supporting Details.**

9. D. A summary is a restatement of the main ideas of a text. Summaries also use different words to restate these main ideas. **Skill: Summarizing Text and Using Text Features.**

10. B. A flowchart is a graphic used to show a sequence of actions or decisions involved in a complex process. **Skill: Summarizing Text and Using Text Features.**

11. C. A bar graph uses rectangles to convey differences between numerical values at a glance. **Skill: Summarizing Text and Using Text Features.**

12. D. A summary that is structurally plagiarized would be ineffective since it would involve rewriting the original words one by one and only changing a few of them. **Skill: Summarizing Text and Using Text Features.**

13. B. Even though the detail about Max setting up the picnic came at the end, it was the event that happened first since he had to have set up before Cynthia came to the park because it was there before they arrived. **Skill: Summarizing Text and Using Text Features.**

14. A. The word clues "had set up" indicates that Max set up the picnic earlier so that it would be a surprise for Cynthia when they got to the clearing. **Skill: Summarizing Text and Using Text Features.**

15. D. Even though the word "beginning" seems like a sequence word indicating something that comes first, in the context of the passage it means they "started to" get thirsty. The other words are sequence words, which indicate the order of events. **Skill: Summarizing Text and Using Text Features.**

16. C. A transition between these two sentences would likely suggest causation. Good choices would be words like *as a result* or *consequently*. **Skill: Tone, Mood, and Transition Words.**

17. C. This passage ironically is an amusing description of an adolescent written by an adult who has enough experience to know that her daughter's huge emotions will pass and the little girl inside her will poke out. **Skill: Tone, Mood, and Transition Words.**

18. B. Authors use irony when their words do not literally mean what they say. The daughter is clearly having an awful day based on her words and actions, and the use of the word "marvelous" adds an ironic tone to the passage. **Skill: Tone, Mood, and Transition Words.**

19. A. This passage establishes irony in the opening sentence by applying a positive adjective, "celebratory" to an ordinary occurrence that is usually negative, such as the banging of a door. **Skill: Tone, Mood, and Transition Words.**

20. A. Effective readers would likely know this is just the life of an adolescent since we have all been through this time in our lives. Entertained would be a more likely reaction. **Skill: Tone, Mood, and Transition Words.**

21. A. The word "instantly" explains how quickly the mother felt "dismayed" but does not transition between ideas. **Skill: Tone, Mood, and Transition Words.**

22. B. "However" and "despite" both indicate a difference between ideas. **Skill: Tone, Mood, and Transition Words.**

23. B. "Furthermore" would be the transition to use as in: *Furthermore, she made a "tsk" sound.* This would show how the author is building on an established line of thought. **Skill: Tone, Mood, and Transition Words.**

24. D. The author's point of view is his or her general outlook or set of opinions about the subject. **Skill: Understanding Author's Purpose, Point of View, and Rhetorical Strategies.**

25. A. Although the author of this passage seems to lean toward the negative impact of technology and youth, the passage does not actually make a clear argument. It only relays the survey results and words from an expert. **Skill: Understanding Author's Purpose, Point of View, and Rhetorical Strategies.**

26. A. The author of the passage is likely concerned with the negative impact technology is having on our youth since he/she only presents the cons of technology. **Skill: Understanding Author's Purpose, Point of View, and Rhetorical Strategies.**

27. B. Rhetorical strategies are techniques an author uses to develop a main idea. An effective way to do this is to appeal to the readers' reason by relying on factual information. The most effective reason is the one about a recent screen time study. It shows that technology use has risen since it's available in so many forms. This is a fact that can be proven. **Skill: Understanding Author's Purpose, Point of View, and Rhetorical Strategies.**

28. A. The passage first reports on the results of a survey about technology use and young people. Greensburg's comments explain the effects this technology is having on young people. **Skill: Understanding Author's Purpose, Point of View, and Rhetorical Strategies.**

29. C. This is a book review. Although it includes some information about the story, its primary purpose is to convince you to read it. This makes it a persuasive text. **Skill: Understanding Author's Purpose, Point of View, and Rhetorical Strategies.**

30. C. Most of the information despite the second paragraph is not verifiable, but the fact that the book chronicles the final years of Audrey Lacoste's life is a fact. **Skill: Understanding Author's Purpose, Point of View, and Rhetorical Strategies.**

31. C. This is a book review. The author includes details about Audrey Lacoste's life to personalize the idea of getting old by telling one individual's struggle. This is meant to appeal to the reader's emotions. **Skill: Understanding Author's Purpose, Point of View, and Rhetorical Strategies.**

32. A. This first statement is an opinion since it reflects someone's beliefs about doctors. **Skill: Facts, Opinions, and Evaluating an Argument.**

33. A. An overgeneralization is a broad claim based on too little evidence, so this would be an example of faulty reasoning. **Skill: Facts, Opinions, and Evaluating an Argument.**

34. A. All of these statements contain beliefs or feelings that are subject to interpretation except the statement about the number of people attending the 2018 London New Year's Day Parade compared to the 2018 NFL Super Bowl. This is a verifiable piece of information, or a fact. **Skill: Facts, Opinions, and Evaluating an Argument.**

35. A. This passage argues that working mothers have it hard. **Skill: Facts, Opinions, and Evaluating an Argument.**

36. D. The writer of this passage makes the assumption that mothers cook, clean, and care for the children. **Skill: Facts, Opinions, and Evaluating an Argument.**

37. D. The author of the passage uses the phrase "the onus ultimately still falls on the working mother." This implies that fathers do not do enough to help out. **Skill: Facts, Opinions, and Evaluating an Argument.**

38. A. This statement takes a complex issue and presents it as if only two possible options are in play. This is an either/or fallacy. **Skill: Facts, Opinions, and Evaluating an Argument.**

39. C. Tertiary sources are very general sources of information that are compiled in a general or highly summarized way. **Skill: Understanding Primary Sources, Making Inferences, and Drawing Conclusions.**

40. B. A biography of a politician would be a historical or analytical account that adds insight on the topic. This makes it a secondary source. **Skill: Understanding Primary Sources, Making Inferences, and Drawing Conclusions.**

41. D. An article on the best farming practices from the turn of the 19th century would be highly outdated. Even if the writer were a professional farmer, the advice presented would likely not be worth following. **Skill: Understanding Primary Sources, Making Inferences, and Drawing Conclusions.**

42. B. Manny is anxiously awaiting the mail. You know this because he "looked out the window," says, "not yet," and bursts "through the door" after he sees the "small, white truck." **Skill: Understanding Primary Sources, Making Inferences, and Drawing Conclusions.**

43. B. Manny opening the cookie jar does not explicitly show that he is eager for the mail to come. **Skill: Understanding Primary Sources, Making Inferences, and Drawing Conclusions.**

44. C. When Stanley shows Manny the envelope from Michigan State and says with a smile, "Is this what you're looking for, son?" it shows that he knows Manny is eagerly waiting to hear from colleges. This proves that he knows Manny pretty well since he knows what's going on in his life. **Skill: Understanding Primary Sources, Making Inferences, and Drawing Conclusions.**

45. A. From phrases like "your children," you can infer that the intended audience of this passage is parents. **Skill: Understanding Primary Sources, Making Inferences, and Drawing Conclusions.**

46. A. The author assumes that many parents have the problem of their children not listening to them or being able to focus well. **Skill: Understanding Primary Sources, Making Inferences, and Drawing Conclusions.**

47. C. The author does not suggest parents do not know how to discipline their children. This article is about setting limits on technology. It is not about disciplining children. **Skill: Understanding Primary Sources, Making Inferences, and Drawing Conclusions.**

Section III. Vocabulary & General Knowledge

1. C. The prefix that means "large" is *macro-* *as* in the word *macroeconomics.* **Skill: Root Words, Prefixes, and Suffixes.**

2. D. The prefix *im-* means "not," and the root word *mut* means "change," so *immutable* means "unchangeable." **Skill: Root Words, Prefixes, and Suffixes.**

3. D. The root *neo* means "new and recent," so a neophyte is someone who it new to something. **Skill: Root Words, Prefixes, and Suffixes.**

4. D. The root that means "city" is *poli* as in *metropolis.* **Skill: Root Words, Prefixes, and Suffixes.**

5. D. The prefix that means "beneath" is *infra-.* **Skill: Root Words, Prefixes, and Suffixes.**

6. D. The prefix *hyper-* means "above or excessively," so *hyperbole* would be exaggeration. **Skill: Root Words, Prefixes, and Suffixes.**

7. C. The root word *circum* means "around," so *circumvent* means "to find a way around." **Skill: Root Words, Prefixes, and Suffixes.**

8. A. The suffix that means "in the manner of" is *-ly* as in the word *courageously.* **Skill: Root Words, Prefixes, and Suffixes.**

9. B. The root that means "cut" is *cise* as in the word *incisor*. **Skill: Root Words, Prefixes, and Suffixes.**

10. B. The prefix that means "across" is *dia-* as in the word *diagonal*. **Skill: Root Words, Prefixes, and Suffixes.**

11. C. The suffix *-cide* means "the act of killing" and the root word *gen* means "race or kind," so *genocide* means many people have been killed. **Skill: Root Words, Prefixes, and Suffixes.**

12. B. The root word *flect* means "to bend," so *genuflect* means "to bow." **Skill: Root Words, Prefixes, and Suffixes.**

13. A. The root *grat* means "thankful" as in the word *gratitude*. **Skill: Root Words, Prefixes, and Suffixes.**

14. C. The root word *trans* mean "across," so *transcontinental* means "across the continent." **Skill: Root Words, Prefixes, and Suffixes.**

15. A. The suffix that means "relating to or resembling" is *-ular* as in the word *muscular*. **Skill: Root Words, Prefixes, and Suffixes.**

16. C. The root that means "life" is *anim* as in the word *animate*. **Skill: Root Words, Prefixes, and Suffixes.**

17. D. The prefix that means "short" is *brev-* as in the word *brevity*. **Skill: Root Words, Prefixes, and Suffixes.**

18. C. The prefix *omni-* means "all" so an animal that is an omnivore would eat both meat and plants. **Skill: Root Words, Prefixes, and Suffixes.**

19. B. The root word *magn* means "great or large," so a magnate would be a wealthy and powerful person. **Skill: Root Words, Prefixes, and Suffixes.**

20. C. The root *locu* means "speak," so a loquacious person would be talkative. **Skill: Root Words, Prefixes, and Suffixes.**

21. B. The suffix that means "a place for" is *-arium* as in the word *aquarium*. **Skill: Root Words, Prefixes, and Suffixes.**

22. D. The meaning of <u>pupils</u> in this context is "the dark circular opening at the center of the eyes." The word "eyes" helps you figure out which meaning of <u>pupils</u> is being used. **Skill: Context Clues and Multiple Meaning Words.**

23. B. The meaning of <u>stark</u> in the context of this sentence is "plain." **Skill: Context Clues and Multiple Meaning Words.**

24. B. The meaning of <u>ferocious</u> in this context is "savagely fierce." The word "attack" helps you figure out the meaning of <u>ferocious</u>. **Skill: Context Clues and Multiple Meaning Words.**

25. A. The word "custom" has more than one meaning. **Skill: Context Clues and Multiple Meaning Words.**

26. C. The word "punch" has more than one meaning. **Skill: Context Clues and Multiple Meaning Words.**

27. D. The meaning of <u>fair</u> in the context of this sentence is "reasonable." **Skill: Context Clues and Multiple Meaning Words.**

28. A. The meaning of <u>dreary</u> in this context is "gloomy." The word "gray" helps you figure out the meaning of <u>dreary</u>. **Skill: Context Clues and Multiple Meaning Words.**

29. C. The word "angle" has more than one meaning. **Skill: Context Clues and Multiple Meaning Words.**

30. A. The meaning of <u>trunk</u> in the context of this sentence is "the torso of a human body." **Skill: Context Clues and Multiple Meaning Words.**

31. C. The meaning of <u>plate</u> in this context is "a small, flat piece of metal bearing a name that is attached to a door." The word "name" helps you figure out which meaning of <u>plate</u> is being used. **Skill: Context Clues and Multiple Meaning Words.**

32. C. The meaning of <u>erratic</u> in this context is "unstable." The word "ice" helps you figure out the meaning of <u>erratic</u>. **Skill: Context Clues and Multiple Meaning Words.**

33. D. The word "match" has more than one meaning. **Skill: Context Clues and Multiple Meaning Words.**

34. A. The meaning of <u>range</u> in the context of this sentence is "an assortment of things." **Skill: Context Clues and Multiple Meaning Words.**

35. C. The meaning of <u>mask</u> in this context is "conceal." The phrase "hiding" helps you figure out which meaning of <u>mask</u> is being used. **Skill: Context Clues and Multiple Meaning Words.**

36. A. The meaning of <u>fluctuate</u> in the context of this sentence is "vary." **Skill: Context Clues and Multiple Meaning Words.**

37. D. The meaning of <u>insatiable</u> in this context is "can't be satisfied." The word "frequently" helps you figure out the meaning of <u>insatiable</u>. **Skill: Context Clues and Multiple Meaning Words**

38. C. The word "channel" has more than one meaning. **Skill: Context Clues and Multiple Meaning Words**

39. A. The meaning of <u>figure</u> in the context of this sentence is "a shape or form." **Skill: Context Clues and Multiple Meaning Words.**

40. A. "Triage" refers to the medical screening of patients to determine their priority. **Skill: Domain-Specific Words: Medical Industry.**

41. C. The root word that means "bones of the fingers and toes" is *phalang*. **Skill: Domain-Specific Words: Medical Industry.**

42. B. The surgeon will excise the patient's appendix. **Skill: Domain-Specific Words: Medical Industry.**

43. C. Enteropathy is a disease of the intestines. **Skill: Domain-Specific Words: Medical Industry.**

44. C. The suffix –*sepsis* means "decay of." **Skill: Domain-Specific Words: Medical Industry.**

45. A. The word *posterior* means "toward the back." **Skill: Domain-Specific Words: Medical Industry.**

46. D. Adding the suffix *pharmacology* would make the word *psychopharmacology* or the study of how medicine affects the brain. **Skill: Domain-Specific Words: Medical Industry.**

47. D. An *orthopedic surgeon* repairs anything that's part of the musculoskeletal system. The prefix *ortho* means "straight, upright, or correct" to refer towards the proper movement of the body which is controlled by the musculoskeletal system. **Skill: Domain-Specific Words: Medical Industry.**

48. A. *Thorac* pertains to the chest, so the patient was experiencing chest pain. **Skill: Domain-Specific Words: Medical Industry.**

49. A. The root word for *reproduction* is *gen*. **Skill: Domain-Specific Words: Medical Industry.**

50. A. The prefix *nephr* refers to the kidneys and the suffix *algia* refers to pain, so *nephralgia* means "pain of the kidneys." **Skill: Domain-Specific Words: Medical Industry.**

Section IV. Grammar

1. B. *Possibility* is the only correct spelling. **Skill: Spelling.**

2. C. *Loneliness* is the only correct spelling. **Skill: Spelling.**

3. C. *Pronunciation* is the only correct spelling. **Skill: Spelling.**

4. D. *Dependent* is the only correct spelling. **Skill: Spelling.**

5. D. President, Is, Elected, By, The, People. Only the first word in this sentence is capitalized. The term president is used generally here and does not need to be capitalized. **Skill: Capitalization.**

6. A. Met, For, Lunch, and Yesterday. The word that begins the sentence is always capitalized. Individual names and familial relationships are also capitalized. **Skill: Capitalization.**

7. C. Of, The, Was, The, Last, Major, Battle, and Of. All names of specific battles and wars should be capitalized, except for short prepositions, conjunctions, and articles. **Skill: Capitalization.**

8. B. Has, Good, and Food. The is capitalized because it begins the sentence. South is capitalized because it is a definite region. **Skill: Capitalization.**

9. C. *I go to bed early so I do not feel tired.* There should be a comma before so as it is a coordinating conjunction. **Skill: Punctuation.**

10. C. *He claimed, "My history presentation was great!"* Quotation marks enclose direct statements. **Skill: Punctuation.**

11. B. *Honesty is the best policy.* All the other sentences are missing some punctuation. **Skill: Punctuation.**

12. D. *Ashley's determined to learn.* Ashley's stands for Ashley is and is the only correct use of an apostrophe in the examples. **Skill: Punctuation.**

13. B. *Matthew* and *Tuesday* are proper nouns. **Skill: Nouns.**

14. B. *crowd* and *speech* are common nouns. There is one more noun in the sentence, *Dr. King*, but it is a proper noun. **Skill: Nouns.**

15. A. *Deer* is both the singular and plural form for the noun *deer.* **Skill: Nouns.**

16. C. *Dishonesty* does not physically exist; it is an abstract noun. **Skill: Nouns.**

17. B. *Her* is a possessive pronoun. **Skill: Pronouns.**

18. B. *Him* is a pronoun. **Skill: Pronouns.**

19. A. *He* is the only subject pronoun listed. **Skill: Pronouns.**

20. D. *Wisely* is an adverb that describes the verb *spoke.* **Skill: Adjectives and Adverbs.**

21. B. *Founding* is an adjective that describes the noun *fathers.* **Skill: Adjectives and Adverbs.**

22. D. *Outside* is an adverb that describes the verb *go.* **Skill: Adjectives and Adverbs.**

23. D. *Perfect* is an adjective that describes the nouns *voice, poise,* and *costume.* **Skill: Adjectives and Adverbs.**

24. B. *The* is an article, not a conjunction. **Skill: Conjunctions and Prepositions.**

25. B. *The table* is the object of the preposition *under.* **Skill: Conjunctions and Prepositions.**

26. D. *What* is not a preposition. **Skill: Conjunctions and Prepositions.**

27. D. *On Saturday* is a prepositional phrase. **Skill: Conjunctions and Prepositions.**

28. A. A complete sentence must have a verb. **Skill: Verbs and Verb Tenses.**

29. D. *Are* is not the correct helping verb to form a question with *take*. *Do* is the correct helping verb, and *will* and *can* can also be used because they are modals. **Skill: Verbs and Verb Tenses.**

30. C. *Had watched* is past perfect, which is the correct verb tense to use here. **Skill: Verbs and Verb Tenses.**

31. C. The subject is *Mai and her friend Oksana*, and the predicate is *love to ride roller coasters*. **Skill: Subject and Verb Agreement.**

32. B. *It's* is a contraction of *it is*. The verb is *is*. **Skill: Subject and Verb Agreement.**

33. B. *He* is third person singular. **Skill: Subject and Verb Agreement.**

34. C. The subject is *my granddaughter*, and the predicate is *was born on January 18*. **Skill: Subject and Verb Agreement.**

35. A. This option would make the sentence a simple sentence. **Skill: Types of Sentences.**

36. B. This is a simple sentence since it contains one independent clause consisting of a simple subject and a predicate. **Skill: Types of Sentences.**

37. B. This is a simple sentence since it contains one independent clause consisting of a simple subject and a predicate. **Skill: Types of Sentences.**

38. D. This is a complex sentence because it has a dependent clause, an independent clause, and a subordinating conjunction, *despite*. **Skill: Types of Sentences.**

39. A. You need to call your mother. It is independent because it has a subject, verb, and expresses a complete thought. **Skill: Types of Clauses.**

40. C. Independent clause. The sentence has a subject and a verb and expresses a complete thought. **Skill: Types of Clauses.**

41. D. Dependent or subordinate clause. The clause does not express a complete thought. When is also a common indicator word that begins a dependent or subordinate clause. **Skill: Types of Clauses.**

42. A. I began swimming every day. It is independent because it has a subject, verb, and expresses a complete thought. **Skill: Types of Clauses.**

43. A. *Found* is the main verb in this sentence; it is not a modifier. **Skill: Modifiers.**

44. B. *Escaped* is the main verb in this sentence; it is not a modifier. **Skill: Modifiers.**

45. A. *Despite their talent and hard work* refers to *the band*. **Skill: Modifiers..**

46. C. *Took* is the main verb in this sentence; it is not a modifier. **Skill: Modifiers.**

47. A. *Snore* is intransitive and cannot take a direct object. **Skill: Direct Objects and Indirect Objects.**

48. B. *Them* is the indirect object for *told*, and *their daughter* is the indirect object for *giving*. **Skill: Direct Objects and Indirect Objects.**

49. B. *Her* is an indirect object in this sentence. **Skill: Direct Objects and Indirect Objects.**

50. B. *The baby* is the direct object of the verb *fed*. **Skill: Direct Objects and Indirect Objects.**

Section V. Biology

1. C. The monomers of proteins include amino acids, which are covalently bonded together to form a protein. **Skill: An Introduction to Biology.**

2. C. There are seven classification systems in the classical Linnaean system: kingdom, phylum, class, order, family, genus, and species. **Skill: An Introduction to Biology.**

3. A. There are several features that scientists use to identify living things. These features include: how living things process energy, growth and development, reproduction, and homeostasis. **Skill: An Introduction to Biology.**

4. B. A control group is a factor that does not change during an experiment. Due to this, it is used as a standard for comparison with variables that do change such as a dependent variable. **Skill: An Introduction to Biology.**

5. B. The hydrogen atoms in a water molecule will hydrogen bond with oxygen atoms. This attraction not only contributes to the charge of water but also the properties of water as well. **Skill: An Introduction to Biology.**

6. C. After pyruvate molecules from glycolysis are produced, these sugar molecules are used to make 2 ATP molecules, 6 carbon dioxide molecules, and 6 NADH molecules. While cellulose is a carbohydrate like glucose, it is not used to produce pyruvate. Electrons are created during oxidative phosphorylation. **Skill: An Introduction to Biology.**

7. B. Prokaryotic cells are unicellular organisms that lack a nucleus. **Skill: Cell Structure, Function, and Type.**

8. A. Eukaryotic cells are known to have a true nucleus which houses all genetic information for a cell. These cells range in size from 10-100mm in diameter. **Skill: Cell Structure Function and Type.**

9. C. Higher order or certain organelles are not found in prokaryotic cells. While these cells contain a cytoplasm surrounded by a plasma membrane, flagella for locomotion, and may have ribosomes, all other organelles are absent. This includes lysosomes, which contain digestive enzymes that break down food in eukaryotes. **Skill: Cell Structure Function and Type.**

10. D. The function of the Golgi apparatus is to help with the processing of proteins received from the endoplasmic reticulum. **Skill: Cell Structure Function and Type.**

11. B. Only found in eukaryotic cells, the nucleus is contained within a membrane called a nuclear envelope. This helps separate the nucleus from the cytoplasm fluid in the cell. **Skill: Cell Structure Function and Type.**

12. B. Autotrophs are organisms that use basic raw materials in nature, like the sun, to make energy-rich biomolecules. Minerals are naturally inorganic. **Skill: Cell Structure Function and Type.**

13. D. All prokaryotes reproduce asexually. This means they require only one parent cell to produce two daughter cells. **Skill: Cellular Reproduction, Cellular Respiration, and Photosynthesis.**

14. C. Photosynthesis consists of light reactions and dark reactions. The dark reactions are referred to as the Calvin cycle. **Skill: Cellular Reproduction, Cellular Respiration, and Photosynthesis.**

15. A. Bacteria like cyanobacteria can participate in a wide variety of fermentation pathways. This is because these organisms are capable of generating energy anaerobically. **Skill: Cellular Reproduction, Cellular Respiration, and Photosynthesis.**

16. A. Prokaryotes like bacteria participate in asexual reproduction. This means they can create offspring using a single parent. **Skill: Cellular Reproduction, Cellular Respiration, and Photosynthesis**

17. C. There are three phases that occur before a cell reaches the mitotic phase: G1, synthesis, G2 phase. A molecule of DNA doubles during the synthesis phase before beginning to prepare for cell division during G2. **Skill: Cellular Reproduction, Cellular Respiration, and Photosynthesis**

18. D. When two sister chromatids come together they are bound by a centromere; this enables them to form a loosely condensed chromosome. **Skill: Cellular Reproduction, Cellular Respiration, and Photosynthesis**

19. C. Cytosine will only bind with guanine, and vice versa. **Skill: Genetics and DNA.**

20. A. The theory of heredity includes the idea that an individual receives one allele from each parent. In doing so, this increases the potential for genetic diversity within a given population. Phenotype determines the physical appearance of a person and all of these traits come from both parents. **Skill: Genetics and DNA.**

21. D. Physical traits such as brown curly hair and green eyes are also referred to as phenotypes. Alleles determine the physical appearance of a person. **Skill: Genetics and DNA.**

22. B. Dominant traits are designated by a capital letter in a Punnett square and a homozygous trait is indicated by two of the same factor, or letter. FF would represent a homozygous dominant genotype and homozygous recessive would be indicated by ff. **Skill: Genetics and DNA.**

23. A. The protein disc that holds two sister chromatids together is what collectively makes a chromosome. **Skill: Genetics and DNA.**

24. A. A single DNA molecule is packaged in a rod-shaped structure known as a chromosome. **Skill: Genetics and DNA.**

25. D. There are four nucleotide base pairs in DNA. These bases form unique covalent bonds with each other. Specifically, adenine pairs with thymine and guanine pairs with cytosine. **Skill: Genetics and DNA.**

Section VI. Chemistry

1. D. The variable that is manipulated, or what is administered to a group as a treatment, is called the treatment group. **Skill: Designing an Experiment.**

2. B. A positive correlation means that one variable increases as another increases. Thus, as more dispersant is added, the amount of oil dispersed also increases. **Skill: Designing an Experiment.**

3. B. A stopwatch is a device used to record time in an experiment. **Skill: Designing an Experiment.**

4. A. Empirical evidence provides data and experimental setups that are repeatable by other people. **Skill: Designing an Experiment.**

5. D. For an atom to carry a negative charge, it must have more negatively charged electrons than positively charged protons. **Skill: Scientific Notation.**

6. D. To find this element, find the element in the fifth row (period) and the fourth column (group). **Skill: Scientific Notation.**

7. B. The nucleus of an atom is positive. It contains protons, which carry a positive charge, and neutrons, which carry no charge. Because the neutrons have no charge, they have no impact on the charge of the nucleus. **Skill: Scientific Notation.**

8. C. For an atom to carry a positive charge, it must have more positively charged protons than negatively charged electrons. **Skill: Scientific Notation.**

9. D. There are 8 ounces in 1 cup. Multiplying 3 cups by 8 yields a total of 24 ounces. **Skill: Temperature and the Metric System.**

10. B. The English system is not universally accepted and consists of a collection of functionally unrelated units. However, it is useful when reporting values of weight in tons. **Skill: Temperature and the Metric System.**

11. D. The conversion between feet and mile is a unit conversion in the English system. Within this system, 5,280 feet is equivalent to 1 mile. **Skill: Temperature and the Metric System.**

12. D. One ounce is equal to 28.3 grams. Using this English to metric conversion factor, 28.3 grams multiplied by 25.0 ounces yields 707 grams. **Skill: Temperature and the Metric System.**

13. D. In a solid, particles have the least amount of energy and do not move as much as they do in other states of matter. The strong cohesive forces between the particles keep them close together. **Skill: States of Matter.**

14. C. If the cohesion between particles increases, then the particles are undergoing a phase change that brings particles closer together. This happens when gas turns into liquid. **Skill: States of Matter.**

15. A. Because gold has the highest melting point, it would take more energy to melt it than to melt lead or mercury. If a substance has a relatively high melting point, it is because the forces holding the particles together are relatively strong. **Skill: States of Matter.**

16. D. In a polar molecule, one end of the molecule is slightly negative, and the other end is slightly positive. **Skill: Properties of Matter.**

17. D. In the lungs, oxygen diffuses into the bloodstream because there is a higher concentration of oxygen molecules in the lungs' air sacs than there is in the blood. **Skill: Properties of Matter.**

18. C. Zinc is a metal and will transfer electrons to a nonmetal, such as sulfur. **Skill: Chemical Bonds.**

19. D. Elements in group 13 all have three valence electrons. **Skill: Chemical Bonds.**

20. A. The bond holds two atoms of the same element together, which means there is no electronegativity difference and electrons are shared equally. The oxygen atoms have the same pull on shared electrons. **Skill: Chemical Bonds.**

21. A. The graph shows that at 30°C, approximately 10 grams of $KClO_3$ can dissolve in 100 grams of water. Half that amount of water (50 grams) will be able to dissolve half the amount of $KClO_3$ (5 grams). **Skill: Chemical Solutions.**

22. C. At 90°C, the line labeled NaCl crosses the 40-gram line. **Skill: Chemical Solutions.**

23. D. A Lewis acid is one way to define the behavior of an acid in solution. These substances are recognized as electron pair donors. **Skill: Acids and Bases.**

24. A. Because the solution has a pH of 3, it is acidic. One characteristic of acid solutions is that they are sour in taste. **Skill: Acids and Bases.**

25. C. This is a neutralization reaction where the acid (H_2SO_4) reacts with KOH to produce a salt, K_2SO_4, and water (H_2O). **Skill: Acids and Bases.**

Section VII. Anatomy & Physiology

1. D. The transverse plane is parallel to the surface of the ground and divides the body into superior and inferior planes. **Skill: Organization of the Human Body.**

2. B. The ventral cavity contains the abdominal, pelvic, and thoracic cavities. **Skill: Organization of the Human Body.**

3. C. Deoxygenated blood returns from systemic circulation through the veins, superior vena cava (upper half of body) and inferior vena cava (lower half of body) and pours into the right atrium. **Skill: Cardiovascular System.**

4. D. A vascular spasm or vasoconstriction occurs first during wound healing. Then, a platelet plug forms, followed by blood coagulation. After a fibrin mesh is formed during coagulation, the wounded site is closed. **Skill: Cardiovascular System.**

5. C. The nervous and cardiovascular systems work with the respiratory system to regulate blood pH levels. **Skill: The Respiratory System.**

6. C. As air rushes out of the lungs, the diaphragm relaxes and returns to its characteristic dome shape. This allows the rib cage to return to its position. **Skill: The Respiratory System.**

7. B. Hepatitis replaces dead liver cells with scar tissue. **Skill: Gastrointestinal System.**

8. C. The sublingual salivary glands are found under the tongue. **Skill: Gastrointestinal System.**

9. C. The ova (egg cells) and sperm are female and male haploid gametes, respectively, and are analogs. **Skill: Reproductive System.**

10. A. The penis, epididymis, scrotum, and vas deferens are components of the male reproductive system; the Fallopian tube, cervix, and uterus are components of the female reproductive system. **Skill: Reproductive System.**

11. D. Tubular reabsorption involves a process during which the filtered fluid contains solutes and water that are reabsorbed into the bloodstream. Nitrogenous wastes are secreted in the distal convoluted tubule to be excreted from the body. **Skill: The Urinary System.**

12. B. Microscopic urinalysis involves spinning down a urine sample so that all sediment particles in the urine are separated from the liquid. These sediment particles consist of cells, such as red blood cells, and other large substances such as crystals and tumor cells. **Skill: The Urinary System.**

13. D. During hematopoiesis, bones generate red blood cells. These cells are associated with various functions in the cardiovascular system. **Skill: Skeletal System.**

14. D. Sesamoid bone consists of small bones like the patella. These bones provide mechanical support and protection. **Skill: Skeletal System.**

15. D. The cell membrane that surrounds a muscle fiber is the sarcolemma. Within this sarcolemma is the cytoplasm of the cell, called the sarcoplasm. **Skill: Muscular System.**

16. A. According to the slide filament theory, after a myosin head attaches to actin it forms a crossbridge. Because of this crossbridge, myosin can pull actin closer to the M-line. **Skill: Muscular System.**

17. A. Skeletal muscle has both thin and thick myofilaments. The arrangement of these filaments within a myofibril creates dark and light bands. These band colors give skeletal muscle its striated appearance. **Skill: Muscular System.**

18. B. Hair is an accessory organ that insulates the body. The hair on a person's head traps heat to help maintain the body's temperature. **Skill: Integumentary System.**

19. A. The hair bulb is found deep beneath the skin's surface under the hair root. Within this region, basal cells are actively dividing by mitosis. **Skill: Integumentary System.**

20. C. The hypothalamus is a structure found in the forebrain and is part of the limbic system. It helps regulate processes in the body using neural and chemical signaling. Chemical signaling via hormones is completed when the limbic system works with the endocrine system, specifically the pituitary gland. **Skill: The Nervous System.**

21. B. Schwann cells are a type of glial cells cell found in the PNS. They produce myelin sheaths that insulate the axon of a neuron. **Skill: The Nervous System.**

22. A. To pass through the cell membrane, the chemical signals must be small and soluble. **Skill: Endocrine System.**

23. D. Melanocyte-stimulating hormones increase melanin production to make skin darker. **Skill: Endocrine System.**

24. C. In this case, the pathogen slipped past patrolling macrophages, the second line of defense. **Skill: The Lymphatic System.**

25. C. The immune system sometimes does its job too well and mounts a major defense against a harmless substance. Such an immune system response is called an allergy. **Skill: The Lymphatic System.**

Section VIII. Physics

1. **B.** Because velocity is a vector, it has a direction and a magnitude. Speed is just the magnitude of the velocity. If the plane's velocity changes but is always in the same direction, its speed (magnitude) must be varying. The speed is a positive quantity, so answer B is correct. **Skill: Nature of Motion.**

2. **C.** In this problem, the object's speed is irrelevant to the acceleration. Only the net force causes acceleration, and it does so regardless of the velocity. Use Newton's second law of motion: $\vec{F} = m \times \vec{a}$, where $\vec{F}$ is the net force, m is the mass, and $\vec{a}$ is the acceleration.

$$\vec{F} = m \times \vec{a}$$

$$\vec{a} = \tfrac{1}{m}\vec{F} = \tfrac{1}{9.7}(3.2, -1.8) = (0.33, -0.19)$$

Skill: Nature of Motion.

3. **D.** Because the ball has no horizontal velocity, just use the equation for height with respect to time. The initial vertical velocity is 45 meters per second, and the initial height of the ball is 0. Also recall that the acceleration due to gravity is 9.8 m/s².

$$y(t) = -\tfrac{1}{2}g t^2 + v_y t + y_i = -\tfrac{1}{2}(9.8) t^2 + (45)t + 0 = -4.9 t^2 + 45t$$

Next, set the height y equal to 0 and solve for t by factoring. $y(t) = 0 = -4.9 t^2 + 45t$

$$0 = t(-4.9t + 45)$$

Note that the ball is at ground level at $t = 0$ (the factor t), but the solution to this problem is for t greater than 0 (the factor $-4.9t + 45$). Set the latter equal to 0 and solve for t.

$$-4.9t + 45 = 0$$

$$4.9t = 45$$

$$t = 9.2$$

The solution is 9.2 seconds. **Skill: Nature of Motion.**

4. **B.** To multiply a scalar and a vector, multiply each coordinate of the vector by the scalar. Thus, $a\vec{u}$ = 3 × (−4, 6) = (3 × [−4], 3 × 6) = (−12, 18). **Skill: Nature of Motion.**

5. **C.** In projectile motion, the distance x an object travels horizontally with time t is $x(t) = x_i + v_x t$, where v_x is the initial velocity and x_i is the initial position. Calling the initial position 0, $x(t) = v_x t$. Because the travel time (t) is 12 seconds,

$$x(t) = \left(450\tfrac{m}{s}\right)(12 \text{ s}) = 5{,}400 \text{ m}$$

For this problem, the initial vertical velocity is extraneous information. **Skill: Nature of Motion.**

6. B. To slide the block, the minimum applied horizontal force must be at least the friction force. Because the friction force is horizontal in this case and opposite to the applied force, it is equal to the minimum applied force to slide the block. Multiply 0.050 by 230 to get that force in newtons: the result is 12 newtons. **Skill: Friction.**

7. D. Friction is generally in the direction opposite to the direction of motion—hence, a car that coasts in neutral, for example, will slow down without changing direction. For a car moving east, the friction force is directed west. The car's speed is unimportant to determining the direction of the force of friction. **Skill: Friction.**

8. B. If the object has a fixed speed greater than zero but its velocity changes randomly, then its direction of motion changes randomly. Therefore, the object is exhibiting nonlinear motion. Because the changes are random, however, it cannot be rotational motion, which is nonlinear but also determinate with regard to changes in velocity. **Skill: Friction.**

9. B. An object in uniform circular motion has a centripetal acceleration equal to $\frac{v^2}{r}$, where v is its velocity and r is its distance from the center. If a satellite is in a circular orbit, its centripetal acceleration is equal to the acceleration due to gravity. Also, r is its distance to the center of Earth. Solve for v:

$$a_c = \frac{v^2}{r}$$

$$v^2 = ra_c$$

$$v = \sqrt{ra_c} = \sqrt{(6.7 \times 10^6 \text{ m})(9.8 \text{ m/s}^2)} = \sqrt{6.6 \times 10^7 \text{ m}^2/\text{s}^2} = 8.1 \times 10^3 \text{ m/s}$$

Skill: Friction.

10. B. The object's velocity, v, is related to the centripetal force, F_c, and the radius of motion, r, as follows:

$$F_c = ma_c = m\frac{v^2}{r}$$

Here, m is the mass and r is the radius of motion. Because the centrifugal force has the same magnitude as the centripetal force, the velocity can be determined given the centrifugal force, the mass of the object, and the radius of motion. **Skill: Friction.**

11. D. The basic qualitative rule of electric charges is that like charges repel each other and unlike charges attract each other. Because electrons and protons carry unlike charges, they attract each other. **Skill: Waves and Sounds.**

12. B. The frequency of a wave is the reciprocal of its period: the time between arrival of successive troughs or peaks. In this case, the frequency is $\frac{1}{25 \text{ s}} = 0.040 \text{ s}^{-1} = 0.040$ Hz. **Skill: Waves and Sounds.**

13. A. Use Snell's law, noting that the angle of incidence is 30° and the angle of refraction is the unknown quantity:

$$\frac{\sin\theta_i}{\sin\theta_r} = \frac{n_r}{n_i}$$

$$\frac{n_i}{n_r}\sin\theta_i = \sin\theta_r = \frac{1.00}{1.30}\sin 30.0° = 0.385$$

$$\theta_r = \arcsin 0.385 = 22.6°$$

Skill: Waves and Sounds.

14. D. The period is the time between the arrival of successive peaks or troughs of a wave. The frequency is the reciprocal of the period: in this case, 25 Hz. Use the wave-speed formula:

$$v = \lambda f$$

$$v = (25 \text{ Hz}) \times (100 \text{ feet}) = 2{,}500 \text{ feet per second}$$

Skill: Waves and Sounds.

15. D. Use Snell's law, noting that the angle of incidence is 15° and the angle of refraction is the unknown quantity:

$$\frac{\sin\theta_i}{\sin\theta_r} = \frac{n_r}{n_i}$$

$$\frac{n_i}{n_r}\sin\theta_i = \sin\theta_r = \frac{2.1}{1.0}\sin 15° = 0.54$$

$$\theta_r = \arcsin 0.54 = 33°$$

Note that when light moves from a material with a higher refractive index to a material with a lower refractive index, it bends away from the normal. When it moves from a material with a lower refractive index to a material with a higher refractive index, it refracts toward the normal. **Skill: Waves and Sounds.**

16. C. Use the formula to calculate kinetic energy:

$$KE = \tfrac{1}{2}mv^2$$

$$KE = \tfrac{1}{2}\left(1490 \text{ kg}\right)\left(26.8 \tfrac{\text{m}}{\text{s}}\right)^2$$

$$KE = 535{,}000 \text{ J}$$

This is the number of Joules the roller coaster car has as potential energy at the top of the previous hill. Then, use the formula to calculate potential energy to solve for height:

$$PE = mgh$$

$$\frac{PE}{mg} = h$$

Then, plug in all known variables and calculate.

$$\frac{535{,}000\ \text{J}}{\left(1490\ \text{kg}\right)\left(9.8\frac{\text{m}}{\text{s}^2}\right)} = h$$
$$36.6\ \text{m} = h$$

Skill: Kinetic Energy.

17. A. The formula for kinetic energy is $KE = \frac{1}{2}mv^2$, which shows that an object's mass and velocity determine its kinetic energy. **Skill: Kinetic Energy.**

18. C. Use the formula for momentum to solve for v. Then, plug in all known variables and calculate.

$$\rho = mv$$
$$\frac{\rho}{m} = v$$
$$\frac{700\frac{\text{kg}\cdot\text{m}}{\text{s}}}{70\ \text{kg}} = v$$
$$10\frac{\text{m}}{\text{s}} = v$$

Skill: Kinetic Energy.

19. B. Use the formula for potential energy to solve. Then, plug in all known variables and calculate.

$$PE = mgh$$
$$PE = \left(7.3\ \text{kg}\right)\left(9.8\frac{\text{m}}{\text{s}^2}\right)\left(1.5\ \text{m}\right)$$
$$PE = 110\ \text{J}$$

Skill: Kinetic Energy.

20. B. Use the universal gravitation formula to solve for r. Then, plug in all known variables and calculate.

$$F = G\left(\frac{m_1 \cdot m_2}{r^2}\right)$$

$$r = \sqrt{\frac{m_1 \cdot m_2 \cdot G}{F}}\text{T}$$

$$r = \sqrt{\frac{\left(2{,}031{,}000\ kg\right)\left(11{,}110\ kg\right)\left(6.67 \times 10^{-11}\frac{N\cdot m^2}{kg^2}\right)}{10.0\ N}}$$
$$r = 0.388\ \text{m}$$

Skill: Kinetic Energy.

21. B. Electric current is the flow of electric charge. **Skill: Electricity and Magnetism.**

22. D. Electromagnetic induction is the creation of an electric force (or electric potential difference) in a conductor by using a changing magnetic field. **Skill: Electricity and Magnetism.**

23. C. Changing magnetic flux through a wire loop creates an electric current in the loop through electromagnetic induction. By moving the magnet away from the loop, the magnetic flux through the loop decreases, inducing a current. **Skill: Electricity and Magnetism.**

24. C. Apply Coulomb's law. The unknown in this case is the distance between the charges rather than the force between them.

$$F_E = k\frac{Q_1 Q_2}{r^2}$$

$$r^2 = k\frac{Q_1 Q_2}{F_E} = (9 \times 10^9)\frac{(5.00) \times (10.0)}{12,500} = (9 \times 10^9)\frac{50.0}{12,500} = 3.60 \times 10^7$$

$$r = \sqrt{3.6 \times 10^7} = 6.00 \times 10^3$$

The objects are 6.00×10^3 meters apart.

Skill: Electricity and Magnetism.

25. C. Use Ohm's law:

$$V = IR$$

$$R = \frac{V}{I} = \frac{120 \text{ volts}}{0.83 \text{ amps}} = 140 \text{ ohms}$$

Skill: Electricity and Magnetism.

CPSIA information can be obtained
at www.ICGtesting.com
Printed in the USA
BVHW082045300420
578097BV00002B/2